Carers in the community: 'Why have you forsaken me?'

DEDICATION

To my Mam, who shared her secrets with me as she battled courageously for many years with her hidden, devastating illness and bore her silent sufferings so nobly.

To Elizabeth, of whom I am so proud, for bravery in pain and struggle throughout her teen years and courage and endurance in coping with her hidden illness.

For without both these persons and the power of prayer, this book would never have been written.

Carers in the community: 'Why have you forsaken me?'

by
Edna Mary Hunneysett

APS

Academic Publishing Services
The Old School, Tollard Royal, Salisbury, Wiltshire, SP5 5PW
www.apspublishing.co.uk

British Library Cataloguing in Publication Data
A catalogue record for this book is available from the British Library

ISBN 0 9537234 7 X

Printed in the UK by Selwood Printing Ltd, Burgess Hill, W Sussex

CONTENTS

ACKNOWLEDGEMENT

I am very grateful to the many people who have helped me in writing this book and, initially, with my dissertation: Petroc, my tutor; carers of the support groups investigated; participants of the interviews; and Ruth who was my companion on the course.

I thank Father Kevin and Josie for support and encouragement; Cath for helpful suggestions and time given listening to me; Father Eddie for kindness and continual interest in my work; and Danny, my mentor, for professional advice, encouragement, painstakingly proof reading, constant support, and invaluable friendship.

I thank my husband Ray and all my children for their interest and encouragement, especially Elizabeth for her patience and technological expertise, for the many hours devoted to reading, correcting and discussing this book of our journey together, as we slowly reproduced our story on paper, and for encouraging me in my determination to bring this topic out of the woodwork when at times I would rather have left it buried.

All persons in this book have been given pseudonyms with the exception of the author's immediate family plus some members of her extended family, all of whom have given permission to be identified.

FOREWORD

When asked to write a foreword to Edna Hunneysett's excellent book, I was initially proud, but then a little anxious. I am a member of the medical profession that, at times, was less than efficient in dealing with the illness of her daughter, Elizabeth. In addition, there were times when the family could have had more care and support in their emotional difficulties. There are many possible reasons why doctors are not good at diagnosing and treating mental illness, despite the fact that it forms a large part of their workload. Perhaps it is the fact that we see so many 'unhappy' people that prevents us recognising those who are seriously ill, or perhaps depressed people are too much of a mirror of our own sadness—and we deny their pain, in the hope that it may go away by itself. I am only glad that we do not treat patients with broken legs and heart attacks in the same way.

The unravelling story of Elizabeth's depression teaches all of us the impact that such illness can have on a whole family. It also demonstrates the paucity of support and services available to sufferers and carers, from the NHS, local authority, Church and wider community. Edna's reaction to the situation can only be described as splendid. The use of an academic study and a carers support group have improved the situation in Edna's locality, and hopefully far beyond, through the publication of this book.

As a non-academic wife, mother and grandmother, it would be easy to see Edna's achievements as extraordinary and unique. A reader who comes to this conclusion is, in my opinion, missing the point: it is Edna's very ordinariness that makes this story and the subsequent research so uplifting. In harnessing a desire to help her fellow man, with her strong faith in God, she has shown that ordinary people can bridge the gap between the spiritual and the secular in the world of healing—and that is a feat to make any health professional feel a sense of humility.

Dr Danny Donovan
Middlesbrough
December 1998

INTRODUCTION

The inspiration to write this book arose out of my personal experience as a carer and from contact with other carers supporting persons suffering mental illness. These experiences triggered my research into investigating the nature of the support available to carers of persons with mental illness, including any Church participation and whether or not it addressed their needs. It was personally important to me to seriously investigate the level of support, and to establish what provisions were available to carers where there is mental illness. By so doing, I hope I may have helped others who may find themselves in similar situations.

As a carer, I found entering the arena of psychiatry and a mental hospital, including meeting with consultants and nurses, an overwhelming experience. This was because of fear, lack of knowledge, and an almost innate shame born of the stigma that can marginalise persons with mental illness. Strong emotions, such as trepidation, self-blame and feelings of guilt, can be experienced when the sufferer is a child of the carer, as in my own situation, and it invariably takes courage to inform relatives and friends of the whereabouts of the person hospitalised. I began by telling friends that Elizabeth was under observation at a hospital as I could not, at first, bring myself to say that it was a mental hospital. I, too, had a barrier to work through.

Over the months, I experienced a great need for understanding of my daughter's illness and for appreciation for myself in my caring role, but felt this was lacking in my own family and in the community. In my church community, prayers were being offered, but did not fulfil the holistic needs I was experiencing and my search for the living human face of God seemed in vain. It is difficult to communicate the depth of my spiritual need in the abyss of isolation and suffering. Eventually I began attending a 'secular' carers' support group, but felt that, although this addressed certain needs, I needed a more holistic approach with special emphasis on addressing deeper spiritual needs. This led me to investigate what support was available within the Church, but I found little. This was mostly because of people's lack of knowledge and understanding of the suffering that mental illness causes, and its effect on carers and families. I began writing about these issues and eventually initiated a Scripture-based support group for carers.

My own experience, gained through working with people suffering from mental illness, medical, health and social services personnel in this field and from listening to other carers, has led to a belief that it is difficult for others to appreciate the impact an individual suffering from mental illness can have on family life. I have come to a greater understanding of just how much mental illness influences all areas of the person's life and the stressful effect this has on those around them.

In the first part of this book, I recount the story of my daughter Elizabeth's teenage years as she struggled with a depressive illness, and of the impact it had on myself and my family. Reference is made to my Mam who also secretly suffered a mental illness. In the later chapters, I relate the outcome of my research into support for carers of people with mental illness and Church involvement, while continuing the account of Elizabeth's progress. My research reflects the literature relating to carers and Church support, and relevant teaching of the Catholic Church on supporting people in need. I review literature on carers, and include some of their personal comments, as well as an analysis of the information gathered from questionnaires completed by carers of two support groups that I attended. There is an overview of the established support in a local community that is offered by the Church to families and carers. This is drawn from the information supplied in interviews with Catholic clergy and a Catholic general practitioner. I conclude with a recap of the findings, together with my own conclusions and personal recommendations.

Section I

1
A CRY FOR HELP

'Can you come and get Elizabeth. She's drunk'. It was Jonathan, our fifteen-year-old son on the other end of the phone.

'What do you mean, she's drunk. She left with friends for a party an hour ago. Where are you? Where is Elizabeth? What's going on?' I was tripping over my words. Ray and I were having a quiet evening together. It was only 9.00pm. Elizabeth, our thirteen-year-old and youngest of our eight children, had asked earlier for permission to go to a party and I had agreed. She was going, she told me, with two girlfriends. There had been no inkling of any deceit.

I grabbed the car keys and rushed out of the house shouting to my husband where I was going. He replied, 'I'm coming,' and locking the door behind him, jumped into the car and we left.

We were not happy. I drove to the venue described by Jonathan. He and his friend were standing on the pavement holding Elizabeth up by each arm. Her two girl friends were hovering about looking very upset. Elizabeth was legless. I looked at her in horror. I was livid. She was thirteen. Who had bought her the alcohol? What had possessed her to drink it?

'Who was it?' I shouted. 'Who is responsible for this? Who bought it?'

'It was him,' stated one of her friends pointing at Jonathan. This was getting worse. My daughter was drunk and my fifteen-year-old son was the culprit.

'You! Jonathan?' I screamed. 'How could you?'

'She asked me to,' he replied. 'I didn't know she was going to drink it herself. She said it was for a party.' At least there was a party, I thought, as if that helped. I piled the girls into the car. The lads said they would walk.

'You won't tell our Mam, will you?' pleaded one of Elizabeth's friends. Apparently only one of them had tried the alcohol and a small drink at that, or so they told me and I chose to believe them. I had enough problems of my own and they both seemed okay. We arrived home and the two friends departed together. I was left trying to make sense of it all.

Elizabeth begged me to let her go to bed but I would not allow her to. She was vomiting.

'You may choke', I said. 'I daren't let you.' I was mortified by the table of events. Nothing like this had happened before with any of our children at so young an age. And to think my youngest son had bought the alcohol for her. Elizabeth looked pathetic sitting with her head over a bowl and a towel on her knee. This was not the time for recriminations. Tomorrow was another day.

* * *

'Why, Elizabeth, why?' I questioned the next day. 'What possessed you?' She looked washed out. Dark shadows under her eyes and a deathly white pallor.

'I wanted to be happy,' she replied. 'Our older brothers and sisters had a drink at Christmas and they seemed happy. I want to be happy.' I did not understand this. She was a clever girl; pretty, tall and slim, with friends and a good home. She was talented on the piano and cello. What does she mean, she wants to be happy?

Elizabeth had shown signs of restlessness before Christmas, complaining of feeling ill and staying off school, which was not her normal pattern of behaviour. She would then complete unfinished project work that had been troubling her, appear better and return to school. During the Christmas holidays of 1991/92 she had asked to visit my Dad's grave. This was an unusual request, as my Dad had died two weeks before Elizabeth was born and she had not asked before. She had always found it difficult to hear about the Grandad she had never met. One day in exasperation, and knowing that I was with my Dad when he died, she had declared,

'I did meet him; I saw him through your tummy button.' I used to try and console her by saying that she was the only grandchild with him at his death. In response to her request, I said I would take her before the end of the holidays.

And so, on one bitterly cold January day, I drove out over the moors to the village twenty miles away where Dad was buried.

There, in the far corner of the graveyard, almost under the hedgerow, was his headstone.

'He does know you, you know. He is still with us in spirit,' I said, as I placed my arm round Elizabeth. She had cried a little and we prayed together quietly in the stillness, sheltered by the hedge, before meandering our way back down the footpath to the car and home. But I pondered. Why had she wanted to go to Dad's grave at this particular time and after all these years? What connection between her feelings and death?

Since the trip, I had noticed that she was becoming a more difficult teenager. Her mood swings, her turbulence and restlessness were increasing. It was obvious to other family members too, as demonstrated at one of our special family meals in February. It was a custom of ours to have as many of the family around as possible on Fridays for dinner. With a large family and different commitments, I had found it more and more difficult for the family to meet up and I felt it important that we spend time together over a meal at least once a week. We used to try for Sunday lunch time, but found Friday evening more convenient, and a special effort is made on my part to provide the extras not normally part of staggered or hurried meals. On this particular occasion, Peter, our twenty-seven year old son, had mentioned football. Some family members are avid Boro fans and the dialogue became a little heated. Elizabeth jumped up and stormed out. 'She's got an attitude problem,' Peter stated. I sighed. She had been particularly difficult lately. Ray, too, had voiced his annoyance to me, as she was continually asking him to take her to school whereas the other children had always walked. This sometimes caused Ray to be late for work, which infuriated him. There were other problems too.

Elizabeth was learning to play the cello and making good progress having passed a number of exams, but she was declining to play at school. She was so stressed about this one morning in February that I wrote a note to one of the deputy teachers asking for her to be excused from playing at the school Mass. I received a phone call from the teacher who expressed disappointment at my decision. After some thoughtful questioning of myself, I telephoned the school and said that Elizabeth was to play her cello. I had come to the conclusion that perhaps I was indulging her. Elizabeth returned this phone call, very distressed and still not wanting to play, but I insisted. She had complied, but very unhappily, and it had shown according to a teacher's comment later.

I was to deeply regret this insistence of mine when I found out the true nature of her problem, but at present I was puzzled and worried. I could not understand her reluctance to play when she was so talented. Was it just school? I did not know, but I consoled myself that, even though Elizabeth seemed particularly demanding, having got to the eighth teenager and with all my experience, I would come through this. We had survived years of coping with the unpredictable behaviour of teenagers. I had loved and been fascinated by the company of the many young adults passing through our home, but I hadn't expected a youngster's behaviour to go as far as this latest episode, i.e. getting drunk at thirteen. This was a new situation for me to deal with.

Three days later, there was more of this mystery. Elizabeth's friends were around, laughing and talking, playing music and having soft drinks. It was good to know they had somewhere to come where they could enjoy being with their own companions. I was in the back room when Elizabeth entered. She put her arms round my neck and began to cry.

'Mam, I don't know what's wrong with me. Why don't I feel happy?' I had no answer. She sobbed for half-an-hour before her tears subsided.

'I'll have to go back in,' she said, 'or they'll wonder where I am.' Only two days later and we had another crying session.

'I know I have lots of friends. I play cello and piano. I'm clever at school. I love my family. Mam, what's wrong with me?' This pattern continued. I could not understand. Nine days after her drunken episode and during one of her crying bouts, which were now lasting an hour, Elizabeth requested that I take her to the doctors. What could I say? How do I tell a doctor that I have brought her because she cries?

Of course. It was like a thunderbolt hitting me. Her drinking spree had been a cry for help. Why hadn't I realised sooner? It was so alien to her character to deceive me in such a way. Now I understood. There was something wrong. She needed help. I booked an appointment. Another day and another spell of crying on my shoulder, while I held her and stroked her hair.

It was on a Wednesday that we nervously entered the doctor's waiting room, took our seats and waited, listening for our call. I was apprehensive. How do I explain? In the surgery, I tried to describe the nature of Elizabeth's symptoms: her irritability, crying bouts, irrational behaviour and feelings of desolation. She also had mastitis. The doctor was sympathetic. He prescribed antidepressant medication and suggested we return in four weeks. I felt that he thought she was suffering pre-menstrual tension. She was a well developed girl, but her monthly cycle of two years was irregular. I panicked inside. I did not want to wait four weeks before coming back.

'May I tell the doctor about the episode, Elizabeth?' She nodded. She knew what I meant.

I felt ashamed and embarrassed having to explain how my thirteen-year-old daughter had been paralytic due to consuming an excessive amount of alcohol. 'But I think it was a cry for help,' I concluded. All my worry and Elizabeth's stress of the previous weeks rose to the surface. We were both crying now. The doctor arranged blood tests for her and asked us to return the following week. Days passed. Elizabeth was becoming more reluctant to go to school. Ray and I were invited out on the Friday evening, but I declined to go. I wanted to stay with Elizabeth, although unable to explain my reasons. I felt anxious, concerned that something was wrong. We spent the evening watching videos. We passed Sunday together on the computer doing my assignment for my distance learning degree in theology. Elizabeth was stressed on Monday when she returned home from school. I found her lying on her bed sobbing into her pillow. I wished I knew what was going on. On Tuesday another visit to the doctor's.

We were both very vulnerable after our visit. This time the doctor had said he would seek advice from a specialist who dealt with this area of sickness. He did not specify the kind of specialist, but I had a foreboding. Did he mean a psychiatrist? I kept my thoughts from Elizabeth. She was upset enough. Again we released our emotions through tears, this time at home. I lived with uncertainty and anxiety over Elizabeth. She visited a friend frequently, but was restless, forever switching from one activity to another, be it decorating, tapestry or baking. I ended up with half stripped walls and a very untidy kitchen. My ex-employer telephoned offering me a shift at the residential home where I had been working part-time, but I declined. I was reluctant to leave Elizabeth.

We visited the doctor a third time. I knew that whatever was wrong with her was worsening, as she was not sleeping properly. She lay awake, sometimes crying and was having nightmares. The doctor now thought it better that Elizabeth and I see a specialist ourselves rather than for him to get a second opinion. He seemed hesitant to say much and appeared rather vague, as if he was reluctant to expand his explanation. I stayed back for a moment as Elizabeth walked out of the surgery.

'Do you mean a psychiatrist?' I asked. He nodded. Although I was expecting this, it was still a bombshell. My worst fears were realised. We returned home, but I did not tell Elizabeth.

Easter came and went. We'd had a hectic weekend with eleven for dinner on the Sunday, but I had been tired due to lack of sleep. Elizabeth had walked into our bedroom in the middle of the Saturday night and was trembling.

'Mam,' she whispered, 'I've had a nightmare.' She crawled into bed beside me and my husband slid out the other side to go and sleep in her bed. She was clammy, her hair sticking to her face. I held her; she was terrified. This became a more frequent occurrence.

Monday, my diary reads: *'Elizabeth not well again. Has mastitis'*. Tuesday: *'Elizabeth cried'*, and later: *'Elizabeth cried 12 midnight–1am'*. Thursday: *'Elizabeth a lot better'*. Friday: *'Elizabeth cried, but all well in the end'*. The following week, the schools reopened. My diary continues. Tuesday: *'Elizabeth went in at 11.10am'*. Thursday: *'Elizabeth rang from school—very stressed. Came home'*.

It was a twenty-four-hours a day worry for me. Broken, stressful nights. Days when she was absent from school, curled up on the settee under her duvet, watching videos while I wrote my essays. We eventually called these days 'duvet days'. She was frightened, of what I did not know, but she needed to be at my side and followed me around like a lost lamb, or alternatively asked if I would sit with her. It was disconcerting. And then there was my Mam.

For many years since my Dad had died, I had puzzled over my Mam. She had begun telephoning me regularly from her flat in a town thirty miles away, often distressed. She was always wanting advice about personal hygiene. It seemed to me she had strange ways of doing things. She seemed to have an obsession about washing door handles. I was so concerned for her one evening after a particularly stressful phone call that my husband and I drove over the moor road to see her. She would only see me. She was reluctant to have visitors. My husband wandered the streets while I consoled her. I did not understand the reasoning behind her obsessions. I let some of my family know she was unwell and my sister Grace took her to live with her in her farmhouse.

Around this time Grace's seventeen-year-old son died in an accident when riding his motor bike. I had sons of a similar age: Stephen, seventeen and Peter, sixteen. Stephen was particularly close to his cousin. They had been spending holidays together since he was four years old. They were like brothers. Stephen had his own motorbike at the time and for weeks afterwards told me that sometimes he could almost feel the presence of his cousin riding pillion. Peter, in the car next to me on the day of the funeral, put his head on my lap and cried. It was a very sad and traumatic period for us all, and an especially difficult time for Mam and Grace.

Eventually, my mother was allocated a warden-controlled terraced bungalow in a village, a few miles away from Grace's home. My older brother, Tony, already lived in the village, which pleased my Mam. I saw her infrequently as she discouraged visitors, but the phone calls continued. It was after many years of listening and trying to help her that I began to realise my Mam had a illness. Eventually I put a name to it. It was an obsessive compulsive disorder, a mental illness.

There is a shame and stigma felt by sufferers of mental illnesses. My Mam was adamant that she did not have a mental illness because she did not identify herself with her understanding of what that meant.

'But Ed,' as she called me, 'people like that are put away. They're not right. I'm fine.' And she was, in so far as she was very articulate, skilled at playing whist, a reader in church and far superior to any of her seven children at doing cryptic crosswords. She acknowledged that her behaviour and rationale in her home were not normal. She had many tablets of soap in readiness for her irrational preoccupation with cleanliness. There were tissue boxes galore in her bedroom, and her mania led her to place each item on her dressing table on a piece of tissue and provoked excessive use of tissues in the bathroom.

This was her hidden illness and she was tortured. Who would attempt to wash a pension book when it had fallen on the floor? Only my Mam, because for her the floor was unclean. Anything touching it became contaminated. And how does one explain the disintegration of a pension book to the lady in the Post Office? Who would balance on one leg in the bath so as to dry the other foot and place it straight into a slipper? My Mam. And woe betide if she dropped the face cloth on the bathroom floor while washing her other foot. Now it was dirty and she would have to hop around for another. Her slippers had glowing strips inside, which shone in the night. She could slide her feet into them without touching the floor.

We shared many laughs over her dilemmas when she had overcome them, but no sooner had I convinced her of the futility of one obsession, than she found herself with a new one.

'Ed,' she would say, 'where do they come from? I didn't used to do this.' It was a continuing battle, but her humour sustained her, together with her incredible faith. She was a delight at times and I loved her. She was adamant that I told no-one.

'I have you and God,' she would say. 'I don't need anyone else.' Many times after an hour of counselling, and it invariably was an hour or more, I would replace the receiver and sigh, 'Oh Mam.' I carried her pain, but loved her more deeply over the years as my understanding of her grew. I learnt to value her friendship and felt privileged that she trusted me at such a deeply personal level, but her conversations with me were exacting and a drain on my inner resources. Now my diary is becoming a repetition of, 'Mam rang; Elizabeth cried'.

My diary begins in May with: Friday: *'Elizabeth not so good at night'*. Monday: *'Did essay all day with Elizabeth'*. Tuesday: *'At the doctor's. Elizabeth off all day'*. On the Friday Elizabeth was going away for the weekend to Wales with the school orchestra. It had been organised some time ago and she had been looking forward to going, but we weren't sure now about letting her go, as she was very unsure herself.

'Perhaps it will be good for her,' I said to Ray and he agreed. It was only for two nights after all. So she went, but on the

Saturday night she telephoned us extremely upset and wanted to come home. We talked at length and she resigned herself to staying.

'I'll be seeing you tomorrow,' I said. 'You'll be all right. Have you friends with you now?' She reassured me that she had and we said our goodbyes, but this was disconcerting for Ray and I. What was wrong?

One Monday a week later Elizabeth was brought home from school very upset. I listened to her pleading for me to take her away to get her better until I could take no more. She began again later in the evening and begged me to do something. She could not face school anymore. I had had enough. I took the telephone directory, looked up my doctor's home number, picked up the phone and dialled. 'Hello', answered the doctor.

'It's Edna. I'm so worried about Elizabeth. It's not pre-menstrual tension. It's not that time of the month. She doesn't want to go to school. She's asking me to take her away somewhere. There's something seriously wrong. I'm very concerned. I don't know what to do.'

Naturally, the doctor was annoyed at being rung at home. 'I'm cooking the family dinner, Edna. I'll contact you tomorrow.' Next day, his receptionist telephoned. We had an emergency appointment in a week's time at the mental hospital's Young People's Centre. My doctor had acted on my plea for help. We were to see a consultant psychiatrist. I now had to tell Elizabeth. I tried to reassure her by saying that a psychiatrist is just a name for someone who specialises in certain areas of ill health, but she knew that psychiatrists worked at mental hospitals. She had heard the jokes and snide comments that people make about the 'loonies' who are sent to those kind of hospitals. Her eyes filled with tears. 'But we will have to go,' I said. 'I want you better and if this is what it takes, we'll have to do it.' What lay ahead?

2
YOUR DAUGHTER IS VERY ILL

The appointment was at 2.00pm. I drove to school after lunch and picked up Elizabeth. We were preoccupied in the car, Elizabeth nervously twisting her fingers as she sat beside me. I was very apprehensive. I had visited patients at the mental hospital a number of times as a volunteer. This time I was going because of my own daughter. My heart was sinking as we pulled up at the hospital. It was difficult to find a parking space. We walked nervously through the door. The Young People's Centre is linked to the main area of the mental hospital by a long winding corridor. We were both feeling anxious as we wandered around looking for someone from whom we could ask directions. It was really difficult to find. An old lady shuffled along the corridor where Elizabeth and I were walking. 'Jesus is going to burn me. Jesus is going to burn me,' the lady screamed. My fear of the unknown, my lack of knowledge, and my almost innate sense of shame born of the stigma that has labelled people with mental illness were giving rise to feelings of nausea.

We back-tracked and took another turning that led us to reception. I tapped on the glass window.

'Yes?' enquired the receptionist pleasantly.

'Elizabeth Hunneysett for Doctor Longman,' I replied.

'Just take a seat please.' Another adult arrived with a teenager. What was her illness, I wondered. We sat in silence. There seemed nothing to say. An elderly lady with a gentle face and kindly disposition, appeared.

'Elizabeth Hunneysett?' My daughter nodded.

'Would you like to come this way please?' I stood up to go with my daughter. 'No, just Elizabeth. You may join us later if you wish. I will come for you.' I sat down again, stunned. My daughter was only thirteen. She was very nervous and vulnerable. I wanted to be with her to support her. Why should I have to wait outside? I found this extremely difficult.

I gazed around. Lurid, dramatic amateurish paintings of strange black and red diagrams and doodles decorated part of the wall on the open corridor. Paintings by patients, I wondered? A poem on how to treat children was pinned to a notice board. It seemed somehow appropriate. My hands were clammy; my body tense. I stood up and took a few steps. How much longer would I have to wait? I returned to my seat. I was in emotional turmoil. It seemed an age since Elizabeth had gone into the consulting room.

'Will you come in please?' It was the elderly lady who had reappeared. I followed her into a large room and was invited to sit down.

'I'm Doctor Longman,' the lady said. She had a quiet, gentle voice. I glanced at Elizabeth. Her face was tear stained. I longed to hug her. The consultant looked straight at me.

'Your daughter is very ill.'

'I know she is ill,' I replied.

'No,' she insisted, 'she is **very** ill. She must come out of school immediately. All her activities must stop'. I tried to take this in.

'Do you mean all as in everything? Even things like piano and cello lessons?' I questioned.

'Everything,' Doctor Longman replied. 'No homework either. I want you to bring Elizabeth here for 9.00am tomorrow morning. You may return for her at 4.00pm.'

She rose and made her way out of the room and we followed. I could feel my heart thumping. My legs were weak. I felt numb. We followed her along the corridor. I sensed her concern and kindness. She must have known what a shock this was to me. She handed me a prescription.

'I want Elizabeth to take this medication. If you go over to the pharmacy at the hospital on the next block, you will be able to get it immediately.' I voiced my thanks and we walked slowly out into the sunshine.

I was in shock. It seemed like a dream, but this was really happening. My thoughts were racing. How ill is very ill? No doubt I would learn more tomorrow. What would I tell people? That my daughter was a patient in a mental hospital? This thought horrified me. The reality was beginning to sink in.

After obtaining the medication, we returned to Elizabeth's school. The head master, whom I had requested to see, was unavailable and we were invited instead into the deputy head teacher's office.

'Hello, Edna. Take a seat. What can I do for you?' I had known James for many years as all our eight children had attended this school. I got no further than an opening sentence when I began to cry.

'Elizabeth's very ill. She can't come to school.' He reached out and touched my arm. I stammered out my explanation. I was so distraught that I was not really able to take in what he said. We went to collect Elizabeth's cello from the music room. The music teacher listened intently. She promised to light a candle for Elizabeth at Lourdes at half-term.

Elizabeth went straight up stairs when we returned home. She dragged her duvet down, put the television on and curled up on the settee. Within minutes she was asleep. Jonathan walked in.

'What's up with her then?' he asked.

'She's very ill,' I replied.

'Is she?' With that he went into the kitchen. Ray returned home much later, tired, ready to eat and have a sleep.

'How did it go then?' he asked.

'She's very ill.'

'How? Why? What do you mean?' And so I told him what I knew, which was very little. He did not seem to understand. How could he? She did not look ill. I went to my friend, Margaret, late in the evening and poured out my troubles returning home at 1.00am. In bed I tossed and turned, reliving the day, wondering what tomorrow would bring.

'Bye,' I shouted to Ray and as he drove away. He had dropped Elizabeth and I at the Centre on his way to work. A nurse met us and introduced herself as Joan. She asked me to wait until she had shown Elizabeth to the day room. Elizabeth had been terrified about coming this morning. On the way to the hospital she had told me all the names she had heard people use when referring to patients in mental hospitals.

'You know, Mam. They get called loonies and basket cases. People say the ones in there have gone round the bend, looped the loop or are daft in the head. These sort of hospitals get called lunatic asylums, the nut houses or loony bins. And now I'm going there', and she had started to cry.

My heart ached for her as I waited for Joan to return. She appeared, sat down, notebook in hand and began questioning me about my pregnancy, about Elizabeth's childhood and her relationship with her siblings and with Ray and I. Had I ever been depressed, she wanted to know? I felt it was like an interrogation. Was she looking for a cause of Elizabeth's illness? Was I to blame, I asked myself? Had I loved her too much? Too little? I eventually walked out of the hospital and down the road, my feet automatically following the path, but my thoughts elsewhere. I arrived home, but could not settle because of worrying about Elizabeth. I tried to study. I shopped. I regularly glanced at the clock but the hands seemed to be moving very slowly today. At 3.00pm, unable to wait any longer, I set off to walk to the Centre.

'Doctor Connolly, the registrar psychiatrist, wants to see you; second door on the left,' Joan stated as I entered the hospital. I knocked on his door apprehensively.

'Come in.' I entered and came face to face with Doctor Connolly. He was a tall man with an authoritative, but kindly presence.

'So you're Mrs. Hunneysett, Elizabeth's mother,' he stated in a softly spoken tone. 'Take a seat please.' It was a small room with a desk and two chairs. Our conversation was lengthy.

'Your daughter is very ill,' he began.

'Yes, I know.'

'I want you to understand how serious this is,' he said. I nodded. I felt he was trying to tell me something without actually saying it. When I asked what was the cause of her being ill, he explained that she had a hormone imbalance overlapping a chemical imbalance, aggravated by her monthly cycle.

'It is a physical illness, but as a result she is in a severe clinical depression,' he explained.

'You will get her better though?' I asked, desperate for some reassurance.

'Yes.'

'And how long will that take?' I continued. I just needed to be reassured that this would all soon come to an end. I wanted Elizabeth well again.

'A few weeks, maybe longer,' he answered hesitantly, holding my attention with his gaze.

He continued.

'I would have liked her to be an inpatient, but because of her age, I think it would worsen the situation. You may take her home, but you must watch her all the time.' He spoke slowly and with deliberation all the time watching me intently. I stared at him. I began to realise what he was driving at. I hardly dare voice my suspicions, but I knew I had to find out.

'Are you trying to tell me she is suicidal?' I asked. He looked very grave and replied,

'Yes, and we do not know her flip-point. You must not let her out of your sight. Bring her back at 9.00am tomorrow.' I looked at him, but could not speak. He looked at me. No more words past between us. We had been talking for an hour. I came out trembling, my legs weak. Elizabeth, on a twenty-four hour suicide watch and I had to walk home with her. I wanted to scream,

'No, no; not Elizabeth; not me.'

We walked home side by side, but my mind was in a turmoil. Would she run under a bus? Is that what he meant? I daren't hold onto her like a child. Elizabeth was giving vent to her frustration and anger at having to go to such a place.

'What good is it?' she demanded to know. 'Why can't I stay with you? It's been awful. One girl flung the pots when we were clearing the table. I was scared. There are kids with behaviour problems, with anorexia, or who refuse to go to school. I don't want to go back, Mam. I feel like a freak in there.'

We finally arrived back home, much to my relief. I telephoned her two older sisters with the news. Throughout the evening tension built up until it became almost tangible. I watched television, but without listening. I was conscious of Elizabeth's every move. Do I follow her into the kitchen, I wondered. What if she picks up a knife? A bottle of tablets? I did not know what to expect. Later after my husband had returned home and I had given him this devastating news, I went to church and told our assistant priest. He said he would pray for Elizabeth in Lourdes and light a candle for her. I slept little that night. I lay awake listening for the creak of floor boards. Would she get up in the night and go downstairs?

Next morning I looked bleary-eyed and had a dull headache. I had to cajole Elizabeth into going to the Centre. Ray said he would pick us up on the way home. Elizabeth was distraught at having to go again. She told me she felt she was being punished for not being normal. She was angry and tearful. I ached inside for her, but had to be firm believing that it was for her own good.

On arrival, I asked if I could stay with her awhile. She was so desperately unhappy and I wanted to care for her. I just couldn't bring myself to leave her in this state. I was given permission. We searched for a piano as she wanted to play. We were told that there was one in the main hospital. We found it, but she only played a few notes. She was very restless. We made our way back and sat in the visitors room. I was loathe to leave her. When it was lunch time I felt I ought to go. She came to the door and sat on the cement step. I walked off and then turned to see a pathetic figure still sitting on the step, quietly weeping. That was my thirteen-year-old daughter. Now I was crying silently; the pain inside me was intense. I did not care about the passers-by who glanced at me, my tears running down my cheeks. I was totally preoccupied with the picture of Elizabeth sitting outside a mental hospital, desolate.

That evening Ray and I had been invited to friends to celebrate their wedding anniversary. It was a small gathering. Ray stayed with Elizabeth. I went alone. I knew I would have to eventually disclose to my friends that Elizabeth was a day patient at a mental hospital, but realised I could only do this gradually because I had to work through the barrier of shame and stigma. I very reluctantly mentioned during the evening that Elizabeth was a day patient at the local hospital complex. This was the statement Elizabeth and I had agreed to, such was my struggle to overcome my built-in fear and ignorance of mental illness and what people might think.

Mental hospitals are seen as buildings that house 'nutters', 'psychos' and 'weirdoes'. Knowing that the psychiatrist had said Elizabeth's illness was physical would not, I felt, make much difference to how she might be viewed. When my friend, Molly, who was also at the celebrations, asked me which consultant she was under, I panicked. She'll know which hospital Elizabeth is in if I tell her, I thought. Such was my need to protect Elizabeth, myself and my family, but from what? Why was I so afraid to tell others? I was not ashamed of my daughter. Was it for myself? Was it because of the culture that so often discounts people with mental illnesses? Would this be the treatment my daughter might receive.

I confided in four parishioners at church the next day. Our parish priest, having heard the news from his assistant, expressed his sympathy. We had a quiet weekend. Only one tearful session with Elizabeth. Being a Eucharistic minister, I was able to bring her Holy Communion, although I was not sure if she agreed to this for my sake rather than hers. She wasn't too pleased with God.

It was now half-term, but Elizabeth had to continue attending the Centre. She was very restless on the Monday evening. She was irrational, argumentative and stormed around or broke down crying. Her anger was released verbally, especially in arguments with her father. She was derogatory in her description of the hospital staff. Some were witches. Doctor Connolly could go to hell. I related this later to the psychiatrist.

'That's okay,' he had said. 'Someone has to be the bad guy. Better me than you.' Elizabeth sobbed in bed that night. I stayed by her side, feeling helpless and inadequate. Words poured from her: pleading for me to get her better; that she was in a tunnel and it was becoming darker and darker as the light was going out; and cursing everyone for not understanding. She was very frightened. She awoke me at 2.00am, disturbed and anxious. Again my husband vacated our bed so that she could be with me. Another very stressful and broken night.

At the Centre the following day, Ray and I sat in the consultant's room and asked if we could take Elizabeth back home with us. Ray was on holiday from school. We reassured Doctor Longman that we could look after her together.

'You may,' she replied, 'provided you bring her here each day to see me. She is very sick.' We reassured her that we would.

Elizabeth was delighted at not staying, but her mood soon changed. She was manic in her behaviour at home. She wanted to go shopping to buy a sewing pattern. We went. Half an hour later she decided to bake and asked for ingredients I did not have. A little later she requested a trip to an outlying village in order to visit the shop there, which sold tapestry wools, and she needed more colours. Her concentration span appeared very limited. My husband and I seemed to be dancing to her every whim. What would she do if we checked her? We dare not risk it. We were unsure of the consequences if she was thwarted. In the evening I sat by her bed hour after hour, being present in her torment as she begged me to take her away to live on our own until I got her better. Ray and I had very little sleep.

Elizabeth had been told by the psychiatrist to keep a diary of how she felt. That same day she had written:

'I feel like a empty shell of myself, not my body, but my person—personality. A transparent chrysalis with no choice of who I want to be or what I want to do. My life has been decided for me, to live everyday as it comes with no meaning to life. I feel as if I am searching for the person I was and want to be—myself, but something keeps pulling it away. I sometimes get a firm grip on it, but it is slipping away. I can see a light at the end of the tunnel, but it keeps dimming and sometimes even goes out. At times like that, I just want to lock myself away in a small dark room where no one can see the person I have become—the person who has fallen into a pit and finds it hard to come to terms with the fall. In this little room I can heal and slowly grow back to the person I was and so long to be; to climb out of this pit. I don't want to die because there are so many things I love too much to leave; family, my music and my friends. Also if I did kill myself I would cause too much pain to the people I love. I feel trapped by an unexplained tormenting presence.'

Wednesday saw us returning to the hospital as requested. Doctor Connolly was angry to learn that we had taken Elizabeth home. He spent an hour explaining how ill she was and that the medical team had considered keeping her in hospital full-time. We told him that the consultant had allowed us to take her home. At this point, Doctor Connolly jumped up and left the room. He returned later, obviously extremely annoyed that Doctor Longman was keeping her word to us. I could understand his concern.

Elizabeth was more cheerful at being allowed home again despite being easily angered and frustrated. She had received a letter from her eldest sister, Kathleen, a home-made card from her niece, Jenny, aged four, and a painting from her nephew, Will, aged three. These gave her much pleasure. I tried to keep the peace between her and her Dad. Late evening, Elizabeth wrote in her diary:

'I have a pounding headache. Also pains in my right foot like in my breasts. I feel quite cheerful, but very tired'.

On Thursday her pain increased. At lunch time she wrote that: *'I have had a lot of pain in my right foot and a small amount of pain in my left. I also keep getting a few pains up and down my right arm. My breasts are still very painful. The pain seems to be more of an ache with sharp point pains'*. Two friends telephoned, which lifted her spirits and she cooked a lasagne for dinner. In the evening I took her to see our twenty-three year old daughter, Jacqueline, who lives locally. Elizabeth wrote:

'I was quite nervous about going out and seeing people because we went to the Off Licence after Jackie's, but I just stayed in the car. I keep getting the same type of pain... and the pain keeps appearing all over my body'. We had tears at night and Elizabeth crept into bed with me, too frightened to sleep alone. Friday showed an improvement, although Elizabeth was extremely tired. Peter turned up for dinner and stayed with Elizabeth after taking Jonathan round to the pub to see his friends, enabling me to go out for a couple of hours with Margaret.

I awoke early next morning, trembling and perspiring, a thumping headache, my clammy hands clenched and with vivid pictures still swirling in my mind from a horrific nightmare. It was 6.00am. I could not get back to sleep. I slid out of the bed clothes, slipped on my dressing gown and crept downstairs. I lit the gas under the kettle. The stress, tension and continuous anxiety of the last months had affected my health. The strain of being Elizabeth's lifeline physically, mentally, and emotionally was wearing me down. I was her life support. I had taken much verbal battering, sometimes continuously for an hour, when she had relentlessly given vent to her anger, frustration and fear.

'And don't interrupt, Mam.' she would say. 'Just listen.' She desperately wanted someone to understand. She released her feelings of despair and verbally hammered family members in her speech to me.

'I have not asked for this illness. I do not want it and my life has been taken away. I want it back. Please get me better.' I was emotionally torn to shreds. I felt a disloyalty to my husband and children whom I could not defend when Elizabeth was so irrational. None of them understood. They had had no experience of an illness like this and were finding Elizabeth extremely difficult to live with. She felt she only had me. I could not let her down.

I had to talk. Who could I phone? A priest came to mind who no longer lived locally. I was sure he would help. It was a bit early to phone but not too early I thought, looking at my watch. I hung on for a few more minutes until 7.00am and having searched through my notebook for his number, I dialled.

'Hello. St Thomas's presbytery.' I recognised his voice.

'I... I... I need to... talk to... someone. Elizabeth... is... very ill.' The words would not come out fluently. I was gasping. There was restriction by a tightening in my chest which increased as I spoke. I was hyperventilating. For fifteen minutes words stumbled out of my mouth, sometimes almost incoherently. Then silence. 'It sounds bad. I'm sorry. Don't you know anyone nearer you can telephone?' 'No,' I answered. Slowly the truth sank in. I was not going to get help from this source.

'I'll be all right now,' I said calmly.

'Sure?'

'Yes, I'll be okay. I'll go and have a cup of coffee.' I put down the receiver. I was unconsciously beginning my search for pastoral support. Isn't that what the Church is all about?

That same evening I brought Elizabeth Holy Communion from 7.00pm Mass, perhaps for my comfort as I felt so inadequate and concerned. I know she was very ill that night. I was everything to Elizabeth, her security, her sanity, her hope and her lifeline. She had written in her diary at teatime: '*I have felt empty... I just feel empty.*'

Later that evening, Ray and I were watching television, but were more conscious of Elizabeth, pacing up and down like some trapped animal, than of the screen. She walked to the lounge door, turned and walked back to the window. She stood gazing out, drumming her fingers on the glass. She no longer seemed to be part of us. Backwards and forwards she stepped. My body was taut. My hands were perspiring. My heart was thumping. I hardly dare breathe. It was like waiting for... for what?

3
I AM STARTING TO BREAK

The drumming on the window stopped. Elizabeth rushed out through the open doorway. I glanced at my husband and jumped up. As I came through the lounge door, Elizabeth appeared from the kitchen and tore upstairs. I ran after her. On the landing she fell to the floor as I reached her.

'Mam, Mam, hold me,' she screamed. 'Don't let me go because I won't be able to stop myself.' She was clutching a bottle of paracetamol tablets. She began to sob loudly, her chest heaving. I wrapped my arms tightly round her. I was terrified. I was panicking inside. I wanted to telephone for help. I dare not leave her. I looked into her eyes, shining black pools, full of terror. Where was she? I prayed and prayed to God to give my daughter the will to hang on to the thread of life still intact.

'Maybe I should take you to the hospital,' I said. Elizabeth looked into my eyes and I could read the horror in her expression.

'Why? Why? No.' The volume in her voice was rising. 'I don't want to go there. You look after me.' It was almost a command and I could not refuse. Who could willingly put their thirteen-year-old daughter into a mental hospital? Who would not respond to such a cry as hers?

We sat at the top of the stairs locked together. I rocked Elizabeth in my arms and quietly sang over and over again,

Be not afraid, a hymn I am familiar with. I could remember the chorus and some of the verse lines. The words are very moving.

Be not afraid. I go before you always.
Come, follow me, and I will give you rest.
You shall cross the barren desert, but you shall not die of thirst...
Blest are you that weep and mourn, for one day you shall laugh...
If you stand before the pow'r of hell and death is at your side,
Know that I am with you through it all.
Be not afraid...

We seemed to be together in an abyss, neither in this world nor the next. I will never forget that look of horror as my gaze met hers. I watched the clock on the wall and could hear its ticking.

We stayed there an hour, me singing and praying, with tears rolling down my face as I gently rocked Elizabeth backwards and forwards, backwards and forwards... Ray came upstairs to see how we were. There was nothing he could do. My dairy reads:

'Elizabeth had a crisis. Suicidal. Loved her'. Eventually with Ray on one side and me on the other, we led Elizabeth back down and into the lounge where the three of us sat side by side. We were very subdued and my arm was around Elizabeth as she rested on me. Her diary reads:

'11.25pm. Tonight I could have killed myself. I just didn't care anymore. I have passed trying and caring'. Later she said she had been in a black tunnel with the walls caving in. She was at the bottom of a dark well and the water was rising.

In the morning Elizabeth was calmer. We had a quiet day gardening. In church, overwhelmed by the experience of the previous evening, I shed my tears. As I walked across the car park a parishioner put her hand on my shoulder saying,

'It's not that bad.' How could she know? I had almost lost my daughter last night. I knew she meant well but I was too raw to accept such a comment. My eyes blurred and I walked away. When I returned home, Elizabeth said,

'I've got my period'. I was pleased and relieved for Elizabeth. We had been through the worst, I thought and reassured myself that she would now pick up.

Later that evening Elizabeth voiced her fears.

'Don't tell them at the Centre, Mam, will you, about last night? They'll make me stay in.'

'I have to, Elizabeth. They need to know what happens when you are at home so that they can give you the correct medication. It will be all right though.' She wasn't convinced and begged me not to tell them. She was so frightened that she would be made to stay twenty-four hours a day and never be allowed to come home. I thought she was overreacting. I felt so sure about this that I continued, 'You hit rock bottom last night, but now you have got your period, you will get better. So I'll be able to bring you home after we've seen Doctor Connolly.' Elizabeth insisted that the only way she would go back to the Centre and let me tell them about her crisis was if I promised to bring her home again after her check-up. I promised as I felt sure that I would be allowed to. Her diary reads:

'I know now it is just a matter of waiting till the pills take effect and till I get better... hopefully from now on I will get better'.

Next day we walked slowly to the Centre, up the steps, down the corridor to reception and announced our arrival. Doctor Connolly appeared and Elizabeth followed him. I had a long wait. He finally came for me.

'Elizabeth is asking to go home, but I've told her she has to stay,' he said.

'But Doctor Connolly,' I responded, 'she is over the worst now; she will be all right at home. I can look after her.' And I explained to him the events of the Saturday night. 'So it will be all right now.'

'But she is still very ill,' he said. He explained that Elizabeth needed to be at the hospital so that her progress could be monitored. 'I'm going to leave you two together to talk this over,' he said and looking at me intently, added, 'and so that you can help her understand why she has to stay.' He walked out, closing the door behind him.

I knew he was expecting me to support him. I was devastated. Elizabeth and I looked at each other, Elizabeth's eyes pleading with me to keep my promise. She trusted me implicitly. What could I say?

'I know I promised you Elizabeth. I'll explain to Doctor Connolly when he comes back. I will not make you stay.'

He came back in and sat down. He was a very gentle man.

'Have you told Elizabeth?' he asked me.

'Doctor Connolly, I can't tell Elizabeth that she has to stay. I promised her that even if I told you about her crisis, I would still be allowed to bring her home. I was sure you would let me. She is over the worst now and I promised.' We discussed this at length and he could see I was not going to go back on my word. He was losing patience with me. He was an extremely busy man and had already given us an hour of his time. He stressed again his reason for keeping her in hospital.

'Very well, then', he said, 'if you take her home we cannot monitor her progress and neither will we then be responsible if anything happens to her.' These were his final words.

I was in personal turmoil. If she harms herself at home, I will be to blame. I knew I had no choice but to comply with his wishes. I looked firstly at Elizabeth's anguished face and then at his, authoritative and serious. The pain was tearing me apart inside.

'Okay', I said 'but you don't know what you are doing to me, doctor,' I stood up and glanced at Elizabeth's tearful face. I felt I was betraying my own self. How could I walk out and leave her? As I reached the door, sick inside, Doctor Connolly added

'And will you call at the nurse's office please, on your way out; Joan wants to see you.' I walked slowly down the corridor and knocked on the door. A nurse opened it and Joan glanced up. She came over to me.

'Would you mind not hanging around please when you bring your daughter. It is upsetting the other patients.' I staggered out, angry, upset, frustrated and hurting.

I followed the pavement with my eyes as tears poured down my cheeks dripping on to my anorak. How dare she say that to me? Elizabeth was my daughter, very ill and I loved her. How dare they ask me not to stay with her? She was only thirteen and very unhappy and I felt I had betrayed her. I raged inside at the seeming futility of it all and was oblivious to any people around or the surroundings. Where could I go? Who could I talk to? I cannot bear this pain inside of me, alone. I am starting to break. There's bound to be others who have gone through this. How did they cope? Did their children get better? But I knew of no-one. There must be others out there suffering. Who are they? Where are they? Somebody help me? I was on auto pilot putting one foot in front of the other.

Eventually I reached Elaine's home, knocked on the door and walked in. She was on sick leave from work. She put the kettle on and passed me her cigarettes and lighter. For two hours I stayed with her. Elaine had been a friend for years and was a good listener. We drank several cups of coffee, smoked and talked. In time my tears subsided and I went home. Later that evening I went out with Margaret and another friend, Paula, who listened to my story. Next morning another struggle.

Elizabeth did not want to return to the Centre. She hated it. I had to use all my parental authority to insist that she go while inside I was bleeding. I was frightened as we walked along that she might suddenly run under a moving vehicle. She was very angry and hurt.

'You don't know what you're doing to me, Mam,' but I did know and it was crucifying me. Her steps became slower and slower as we approached the hospital. What am I doing to her? How can I be so cruel?

'You know, I hate that place, Mam. Why can't I stay at home with you? I don't do anything there.' We finally arrived and I left with both of us in tears. When I returned at 4.00pm, I saw Elizabeth wandering around aimlessly.

'Doctor Connolly,' I said, 'she's like a zombie on that medication' and inside I was screaming: 'I can't take any more of this'.

'Yes I know. I'm sorry,' he replied. We are trying to get the right balance. It is difficult, but I agree, the treatment is too severe.' The next day I had a long unscheduled talk with him. He was really kind and helpful. Elizabeth no longer had to take her midday tablet. She was on various medications including Oil of Evening Primrose, antidepressants, painkillers, sleeping tablets and medicine to treat physical ailments. Her whole system seemed to be breaking down. On Thursday morning at home Elizabeth delayed every action and was late arriving at the Centre. She wrote in her diary: *'9.20pm I just want my life back. I've had enough, I hate the Centre.'* Friday was even worse.

'Jonathan, I cannot find her,' I shouted. I rushed upstairs and downstairs, in and out of rooms. I checked the back lobby and our large back garden with its six foot high privet hedges. 'Elizabeth,' I yelled. I ran to the bottom of the garden where we had a large walk-in air-raid shelter. It was cold inside. There were a few empty coke tins and some wrapping papers among the cobwebs and scurrying spiders, but no Elizabeth. I was panicking inside as I ran back to the house. I checked her bedroom again. 'Jonathan,' I shouted again, 'she's done a runner.' I was so scared. My imagination was running wild. Is she already mangled under a bus? I rushed back down our long central corridor to the tiny front lobby and opened the door. No Elizabeth. I flew back again and in desperation even looked in the cupboard under the stairs. Huddled on the floor, among brushes, shoes and the vacuum cleaner, was Elizabeth. 'Elizabeth, don't do this to me,' I pleaded. She wrote in her diary that night:

'I felt like running away and never coming back. I was going to, but Mam stopped me'.

We struggled through another weekend with Elizabeth alternating between being depressed, happy and restless. I wrote in my diary on Monday: *'Took Elizabeth—very reluctant, hurt and angry—to the Centre'*.

Elizabeth's diary reads: *'10.46pm I felt bad this morning because every time I have to go back there, it is like the first time'*. It continues: *'I read over my diary from January to the beginning of May and it was written on a few occasions that I felt suicidal and almost everyday that I felt down and depressed. I felt good about myself today, but all I want is my life back'*. It was when she showed me her diary that I realised the reason for her reluctance to play her cello at school. She had written that she felt suicidal, but had not told me at the time. She said she had not known whether she was supposed to feel like this and thought it might just be how one feels at puberty. How I regretted insisting on her playing at that school Mass.

As well as keeping a diary, Elizabeth had a chart to colour in daily. There were three blocks to each day for mornings, afternoons and evenings. She had to colour in the extent of how depressed she was; the more colour, the worse her depression. Today she had coloured half black for the morning with the afternoon and evening completely black. On Tuesday there is even more black colour showing and Wednesday's blocks are almost all black. She is a very sad, sick girl.

Each day passed. A struggle in the mornings; some happy moments and some tears; and constant anxiety when I leave her. I wave and she waves from the step. I turn my back and walk to the car heavy-hearted. On Thursday Elizabeth seemed a bit brighter. I felt I could leave her in the evening to visit Paula. We had hardly begun chatting when the telephone rang.

'It's for you, Edna,' Paula said, handing me the phone. I took the receiver. 'Hello'.

'Ed, it's Ray. She's gone.'

'Gone? What do you mean, she's gone? I left her with you. Can't you just look after her for once?' My voice was rising. I was angry and concerned. 'I must go,' I said to Paula. 'Elizabeth's gone.' Paula hugged me.

I hurried down the road, across the Common and up our road. Ray was checking Elizabeth's friends by phone when I arrived.

'Why couldn't you watch her?' I raged. I had little patience with anyone. Elizabeth told me later that she had felt very depressed. She had sneaked out and walked across the front garden and through the hole in the hedge so as not to have to pass by the window and be seen. She had walked a long way—just walking and crying and had arrived at a friend's house. So we found her safe. Her diary reads: *'Today I have felt worse and worse. Tonight I know why I feel down, but while I feel like this I don't want to live through it. I still want to live, I have lots of reasons to live. I just would rather be locked away in a little room 'til I get better'*.

I sat by Elizabeth's bed late that night. She had requested a move to the smallest bedroom. She thrashed around, her arms and legs flailing.

'Get me better; why doesn't someone get me better. Take me away, Mam. Just you and me. We'll live on our own out in the country 'til I get better.' She was in pain physically, mentally and emotionally. I could do nothing for her. I knelt by her bed and stroked her hair, listening to her pleadings and sobbing. Elizabeth drew pictures trying to express her pain. One is of a large eye and inside the pupil she has drawn a heart symbolising her life. It is practically all black indicating how depressed Elizabeth was. A minute white crescent shape on the heart represents the tiny bit of light left in her life. She hurts so much that the heart sheds many tears forming a blue sea. The intensity of her pain and suffering is represented by the red, orange and yellow flames shooting out from the sea. What could I do for her?

In the early hours of the next morning I was tossing about in bed frantically trying to think of how I might take Elizabeth away for a short spell. She asked me incessantly to take her away and I thought a short break might be beneficial for her. I rang my sister Grace on the farm before Elizabeth left for the Centre. Grace was happy to oblige. I warned her that Elizabeth may not be sociable as she was hesitant to go out at all and when out with Ray or myself was reluctant to get out of the car. At least we could go on long walks together, I thought. Later I telephoned Doctor Connolly at the hospital to sanction our trip. He was very good to me. If I was unable to speak with him, he would always return my call as in this instant. He was compassionate when I expounded my reason for phoning, but declined my request after learning that my sister lived twenty miles away.

'I want her near this hospital', he explained.

When I returned to the Centre, I had the difficult task of relating this to Elizabeth and consequently of disappointing her. My ex-employer telephoned again wondering if I was now able to return to work, but I explained that I could not leave Elizabeth. Elizabeth told me at teatime that she had had a long conversation with Doctor Connolly and Joan. My diary reads:

'Did not tell me much. I am stopping asking'. She did inform me that she had been told we were too close to each other and that she had to distance herself from me. Elizabeth was angry about this.

'They don't realise that you have a good relationship with all your children, Mam. They have such a cheek telling me to separate myself from you.' I kept an appointment with my own doctor. I walked into his surgery and said,

'I'm not ill but if I don't talk to someone I will be.' My diary reads: *'he was very kind'*. I went out with friends at night, but have written: *'feel some are sick of me talking about Elizabeth, even Ray'*.

I was troubled on Saturday. I had a deep need for understanding and empathy. I took the car and drove to a neighbouring parish with the intention of going to the sacrament of reconciliation. Deep down I knew it was a ploy to tell the parish priest whom I had known for years, of my pain. I was again unconsciously searching for pastoral support. During the course of our dialogue, face to face at my request, I broke down and poured out some of my troubles.

'Aren't you getting any help?' he asked.

'No,' I replied. He said no more about it, but I had hopes that he might do something. Maybe he'll get someone to come and see us. As days went by and nothing materialised, I realised my hopes were futile. After all, I told myself, he wasn't my parish priest. He has his own parishioners to care for. I would just have to keep going.

Elizabeth was very reluctant to go to the Centre on Monday morning and I had no car. Who could I get to take her? I rang Ben, a family friend and neighbour, who was always willing to help. When he answered the phone, I asked him if he could take her for me. I found him sympathetic and shortly afterwards he pulled up outside our house. I told him Elizabeth would show him where the Centre was. I didn't feel so good. Life seemed such a struggle. My diary reads: '*I cried. Slept. Shouted at Jonathan and Ray. Feel I want to cry*'. The colour on Elizabeth's chart for the day was almost all black. When will all this trauma end? It just seems to go on and on.

On Tuesday, I dropped Elizabeth off at the Centre, came home and hung out the washing. Early afternoon after having been for the shopping, I was folding the clean washing when I heard the front door open. 'Hello,' I heard a voice call. I looked up and there stood Elizabeth, smiling. How had she got here and why?

4
EDNA, YOU NEED HELP

'What are you doing here?' I asked Elizabeth, amazed at seeing her.

'They've discharged me. They said I could come home. I'm now an outpatient', she replied. I was stunned at first and then angry. To think that she had been allowed to leave the hospital and walk home on her own. Surely someone ought to have telephoned me. Was this a practise at mental hospitals, to allow patients as young as thirteen to come home alone? I'm her mother and no-one had bothered to let me know. Don't I count for anything? I'm the one who looks after her. 'Why didn't you ring me? I would have come for you. I don't like to think of you walking home on your own.'

'I did ring, Mam, because they told me to, but Jonathan answered and said you were at the shops. So I told him it didn't matter. I wanted to surprise you. I told them that somebody was in at home and I just thought I'd come.'

She was delighted to be home and at not having to stay at the hospital all day. I was pleased for her thinking this must mean she was a lot better, but I felt confused and ill at ease about how this had happened. Later that evening Ray and I decided to go out for an hour. Jonathan was at home with Elizabeth. We had only walked halfway down the road when I heard running footsteps. It was Elizabeth.

'I don't want you to go. I'm frightened to be on my own with just Jonathan'. We turned back. She was obviously far from well.

Doctor Connolly telephoned me the next morning and explained about Elizabeth's discharge. The medical team knew she was unhappy at the Centre and that she would be well looked after at home. Consequently, they had decided that it was in her best interests for her to be an outpatient with a weekly check-up. Doctor Connolly added that if I was at all worried or needed advice, I could ring him at the Centre. More than ever I felt her life was in my hands. In the following days, Elizabeth argued with

Jonathan and had verbal battles with Ray. We walked on egg-shells. I was pulled in all directions—loyalty to my husband, understanding to my son and care for my daughter. Jonathan decided to go and spend a week with his oldest sister, Kathleen, and his young niece and nephew, in Reading. He had finished his GCSE exams and was finding Elizabeth difficult to live with. Elizabeth was distraught at this. She wasn't well enough to go and she wouldn't even have Jonathan's company. She blamed her illness.

On Saturday morning I went to Mass, sat by myself and let the tears flow, which helped release pent-up tension and anxiety. I tried not to cry at home because Elizabeth would feel she was the cause of my pain. Sister Marie, a nun whom I knew, sitting in front of me, turned round and asked what was the matter. She was very sympathetic when I told her. She knew Elizabeth.

'Let me come and see her, Edna,' she said. As she didn't belong to our parish, I didn't want to trouble her, but she insisted and I said she could come.

This was the first time a nun or priest had offered to visit Elizabeth and I was so glad. It helped me to feel it was all right to expect support from the Church, even though this was as much a personal visit by Sister Marie because Elizabeth had attended her nursery school. A little later that morning, Sister Marie came and spent a short time with Elizabeth. On leaving, she said she would come again. At least, now, I felt someone from the Church had recognised my need, although I would still have liked a priest to come. To me, this would have been an acknowledgement of the gravity of Elizabeth's illness and would have meant that she was being treated like any other seriously ill church-going person, and that the family was being given pastoral support.

Elizabeth cried on and off most of the day and her behaviour was very erratic. Hour after hour passed. I didn't know what to do or whether to get help. At 11.00pm I rang the doctor on call because I didn't feel I could get through the night with her in such a state. The doctor arrived and listened to my concerns. He shook his head saying,

'I'm sorry. I can't prescribe anything for your daughter because she is already on medication.' I thanked him for coming out so late and showed him to the door. We were on our own.

Over the next seventeen days, Elizabeth did not get out of bed except for the toilet. I brought her meals and stayed with her. She was frightened of the world outside her bedroom, frightened of its emptiness and of her own feelings. She did not even get up when her brothers and sisters came to wish her a happy fourteenth birthday. They went upstairs and sat by her bed. Sister Marie came again especially to see Elizabeth for her birthday, and spent time talking with her. I was standing on the landing when she came out of Elizabeth's room. She stopped to speak to me quietly. 'Edna, you need help. You can't deal with this alone.' She had recognised that Elizabeth was seriously ill and realised the effect that this was having, and would continue to have on me and our family, but I hadn't fully grasped the situation and wondered at the time why she thought I would need help. I was soon to find out.

My family weren't convinced of Elizabeth's illness.

'What's she doing in bed, Mam?', asked one of my daughters. 'You look tired out.'

'She's very ill,' I replied.

'No she isn't Mam, but then you always did spoil her with her being the youngest.' Ray, too, was bothered.

'I don't think it's right a healthy girl like her lying in bed all day. She should get up and do something.' This was awful for me. Even my family weren't supporting me. But I had to be with Elizabeth and defend her. She didn't have anyone else. I felt so alone. I felt my family thought it was just me fussing. My friends too. One who visited told me I shouldn't jump to Elizabeth's call, but let her wait

'And I wouldn't let her talk to you like that either,' she said. But I wanted to give Elizabeth any little comfort possible. She was so unhappy. I felt I was becoming more alienated from Ray and the other children. Why didn't someone see what I was going through? No-one seemed to understand.

'All right, then,' I said to Ray one day. 'I'll ring Doctor Connolly and ask him.' I was beginning to think maybe I was wrong. I rang the Centre and explained to the doctor my family's concerns. 'Am I wrong, doctor?' I asked.

'No, you are right', he replied. 'It's her illness. She's in a severe clinical depression. You just keep loving her and we'll get her better.' I was reassured. I suppose it was difficult for anyone who had not had any experience of this kind of illness to understand, especially when Elizabeth had no obvious physical symptoms.

Elizabeth and I had a double appointment with the dentist on the Friday, but I went alone. 'And how are you?', the dentist asked. I talked for the next fifteen minutes pouring out my tale of woe. Later in the day, the dental nurse who had listened to my story, arrived at our house with flowers and a card.

'Are they for Elizabeth?' I asked.

'No, they're for you because I was so touched by what you said. You deserve them.' I thanked her and my eyes filled with tears. I was so moved by her thoughtfulness and compassion. In the evening, Elizabeth had another long crying session. Would it never end?

At church the next morning, I told a visiting priest my troubles and as usual, the tears flowed. I was totally preoccupied with Elizabeth and how ill she was. The priest was sympathetic and wrote her name down.

'I will pray for her,' he said. This was the fifth priest I had confided in, but none had offered to visit her. Maybe they thought the chaplain to the mental hospital was visiting Elizabeth, but she wasn't even visited in hospital. Many months later I learned that in some hospitals the denomination of patients is not disclosed to chaplains, as it is deemed to be confidential information. The Catholic chaplain had been unaware that Elizabeth had been in the mental hospital, whereas at the hospital on the adjoining site, chaplains have access to names of patients belonging to their respective denominations. My parish priest did ask after her at evening Mass.

Another week passed with no change. I rang the Centre to speak to someone for reassurance because I was so worried about Elizabeth. In the evening Peter, my son, and his wife offered to stay with Elizabeth to keep her company while Ray and I went out, but even when socialising, all I seemed to talk about was Elizabeth. On Saturday, she was brighter and luckily, two friends called to see her, which made her feel a bit more normal.

We spent hours listening to Elizabeth when she eventually came down stairs. She released her anger amid tears by raging and storming around before breaking down and sobbing. We felt inadequate and pained and powerless to do anything. Ray reacted by going for walks around the streets to compose himself. He told me that he felt for Elizabeth, but did not understand. He argued with her and tried to put forward a different point of view, but to no avail. Elizabeth would berate him before flooding into tears and rushing upstairs. I would go after her and Ray would follow trying to put matters right . The saga was relentless. Although I knew Ray was struggling, it was Elizabeth I felt for most. She was the one who was ill.

I was still anxious for some pastoral support and when Ben rang to see how things were, I asked him if he knew the chaplain to the mental hospital. He did and he said he would speak to him when next he saw him. I wanted a priest to visit Elizabeth as I know giving the Sacrament of the Sick to ill people is an important ministry of the Church. I was sure that had Elizabeth's illness been a serious visible one, we would have had a priest visiting and I could not understand why no-one had come. I felt neglected and thought that there should be more pastoral support than promises of prayers. Maybe mental illness wasn't seen as being serious.

I was in a terrible dilemma because I had to make a decision about whether or not to go to Birmingham on a week's summer school, an essential part of my degree course. I desperately wanted to go, but should I leave Elizabeth? I asked Doctor Connolly's advice. He seemed uncertain in his response.

'Is it very important that you go?'

'It is important to me', I said. 'I will miss an awful lot of lectures if I don't go. My daughter Stephanie, who is twenty-seven, will be at home for a few days and she will be a help and distraction for Elizabeth, but obviously I won't go if you think that unwise. You know I'll do anything for Elizabeth.' He nodded, listening.

'Maybe it will be good for both of you,' he said.

'Also Doctor, about Elizabeth. She is still very ill. I know she is no longer suicidal, but otherwise she's no better, is she?' He agreed and said that he had tried on his own, but now realised he needed more help to sort out Elizabeth's hormones.

'I will get an urgent appointment for Elizabeth to see a consultant gynaecologist and I think it's okay for you to go to your summer school provided you are happy with your arrangements for Elizabeth.'

I had nightmares that Wednesday night. Thursday my diary reads:

'Could scream at Elizabeth and Jonathan arguing. Spent time with Elizabeth. Elizabeth cried—frightened. Slept with me'. And what should I do about Birmingham? Early Friday, I made a decision; I would go. Elizabeth could ring me every day. If she deteriorated, I could come home. I went down town and bought my bus ticket. When I got home, Jonathan had a message for me. Elizabeth had to be at the nearby hospital for 12 noon to see a consultant gynaecologist. That was an emergency appointment as it was only two days since we had seen Doctor Connolly. I was delighted this had happened before I went to Birmingham.

We went to the hospital and were shown into a cubicle where we waited until the consultant came in. He was kind and gentle.

'So you've been wanting to harm yourself, have you?' he asked Elizabeth. She nodded. He examined her, asked questions about her monthly cycle and prescribed hormone controlling medication and advised a further appointment. We were immensely grateful to him. Ray picked us up. We called in at home for my bags and went straight to the station to catch the bus. Before getting on, I hugged Elizabeth and Ray and reminded them of Elizabeth's appointment the following Wednesday. I knew Elizabeth didn't want me to go.

'I'll ring every day,' I shouted, as the bus started pulling out of the station. 'Look after her, Ray.' I watched them waving until they disappeared out of sight.

The students on the BA degree course were of all ages and from varied backgrounds. Some were academics and others, like me, had never studied at higher level, but as a group we were bonded, not in the sense that we had known each other for years, but at a deeper more spiritual level. This sprang from our wanting to study theology and deepen our faith knowledge. I arrived in time for a cup of tea before evening dinner and the first lecture. As soon as someone asked me how I was, I burst into tears and began my tale of woe. The students were wonderful. Word soon got round about Elizabeth. One student announced in chapel that evening that 'night prayers tonight are especially for Edna's daughter, Elizabeth.'

I felt listened to and found the understanding that I had needed so much. I sensed that the students cared about me and my daughter, and that I was believed in without any questions or advice giving. I felt loved by this small community at a spiritual level and through their personal approach. It seemed strange that I had travelled all the way to Birmingham to experience this kind of support.

Every night I rang home where Elizabeth was struggling trying to keep going, knowing how much my studies meant to me. She rang me often, but sometimes it was during lectures and I had to return her call at a later time. She had become desperate one night and rang in the early hours of the morning, but no-one had answered. It was difficult for both of us. I arrived home the following Friday to be greeted with bear hugs as I stepped down from the train, and Elizabeth cuddled up to me as we sat together in the car going home. It was good to be back, but would it be any better? Would it just all start again?

Although Elizabeth was still very unwell, it had been suggested to us that she put in a day or two at school at the end of term to prepare her for her possible return in September. She cried on the Sunday, the day before going in. She was very apprehensive about facing people. On Monday she managed to stay at school for an hour, but it had been an ordeal for her just walking through the school doors and facing her peer group. I made an appointment to speak with the head master the following day, the last day of term, as I wanted to have a chat about Elizabeth and, although we hoped she would be able to cope with school, we weren't sure of what the future might hold. Elizabeth stayed longer at school on the second day, but was very distressed at home later. Twice I found her on her bed sobbing. It was harrowing. I told her I would do anything to make her life more bearable, to give her some happiness. Late that evening she came down stairs.

'I've been thinking, Mam. I know what I'd like you to do for me. I'd like you to take me to Lourdes so that I can go to the Grotto and ask Our Lady to get me better.'

5
LOURDES: SHE DOESN'T HAVE A BADGE

Lourdes. How do I get Elizabeth to Lourdes? I had been once several years ago and came home feeling refreshed, renewed and at peace. Elizabeth had remembered this. Now she wanted the same.

'It's my last hope, Mam,' she said. 'I've tried everything else.' I rang Ben because he had many contacts at home and in Lourdes. The next morning he rang me back to ask if we could be ready the following Monday morning at 3.00am. A coach was passing through on its way to Liverpool to pick up pilgrims going on the Liverpool diocese's annual pilgrimage.

I telephoned Doctor Connolly to ask his permission because Elizabeth was still very sick. He asked me to take her to the Centre the next morning for a check up. He sanctioned the trip.

'If that's what you want,' he said.

'It's what Elizabeth wants,' I replied.

'I won't be seeing you again,' he added. 'My six months is up and I move on.' I was dumbfounded.

'How can you go? You have just got me through the worst trauma of my life and now you are going?' He had always been patient and kind to me and given me time. I had such faith in him. I spontaneously put my arms round him and thanked him. Elizabeth smiled at his look of surprise.

'That's our Mam,' she said. 'She hugs people.'

On Friday I went down town and queued at the post office to get passports. On Sunday a kindly parishioner gave me twenty pounds towards expenses and a nun with her, promised prayers for Elizabeth. Our parish priest generously gave me fifty pounds.

'It's my personal money', he said. He was so kind and compassionate. I was very touched at being offered this financial support and the prayers. At 2.00am I was woken by the alarm ringing. I peeped through the curtains. It was dark outside. I woke Elizabeth, dressed myself and went down stairs to make a cup of tea. Ray walked with us to the top of our road where Ben was waiting. Elizabeth was shivering and I wrapped a blanket round her. The coach arrived. I thanked Ben and hugged Ray. We climbed on. The bus pulled away and we waved until they were out of sight.

It was my birthday, but this seemed an irrelevant detail in my life. No-one remembered at 2.00am. I spent my birthday travelling on a coach. Our coach filled up in Liverpool and off we went down the country, across the ferry and into France. We arrived at the hotel in Lourdes on Tuesday afternoon, both of us very tired. Elizabeth had enjoyed the journey when awake, but spoke to no-one and, when off the coach, stayed close to me. A lady sitting opposite had asked, 'Is she ill?'

'Yes.'

'I thought so,' she had said. 'It's the way she is with you.' I said no more.

It was a lovely hotel. We had a bedroom with a balcony overlooking the river. After the evening meal, Elizabeth went to bed and I told her I would lock the door if I went out. She was exhausted and fell asleep. I decided to venture out and visit the Domain. I was longing to walk in the torch light procession. It was very warm and the streets in this part of Lourdes were full of people laughing, chatting and sometimes singing. The whole place was alive. I made my way through the crowds and went into a shop to buy two candles with holders to carry in the procession the following day, one for me and one for Elizabeth. I was so looking forward to showing her around and joining in all the daily Masses and processions.

I reached the gate to the Domain and began to head across the square that is dominated by the huge statue of Our Lady in the centre. I viewed the enormous Basilica to the right of me and could see the Grotto in the distance. It was good to be back. As I approached the starting point of the procession I noticed the swift flow of the river as, from over the bridge, people were thronging to join the other pilgrims congregating from all sides. I knew no-one, but tagged along and slowly the procession began to move.

It was a spectacular sight. There were hundreds of wheelchairs being pushed by nurses in uniform. I noticed some of the youth of the Liverpool Diocese in bright yellow tee-shirts, helping. There was a great variety of large banners being carried, each denoting pilgrims from different countries. The procession was about a dozen deep and stretched as far as the eye could see, and they were still coming. People numbering hundreds were raising and lowering lit candles to the music and singing. Prayers and hymns were alternated and a number of languages were used so that eventually we could sing and pray in our own tongue. But I felt ill at ease. Maybe I should not have left Elizabeth. It was beginning to dawn on me that maybe this Lourdes for me was to be with Elizabeth twenty-four hours a day.

* * *

'Just look at that, Mam,' said Elizabeth pointing to a glass statue of the Virgin Mary with a halo of stars flashing on and off like some Christmas decoration. There were shops galore full of every possible size and design of medals, statues, crosses, rosary beads, plaques and other such memorabilia. We had been up since 8.30am and spent the day browsing round the shops. Elizabeth loved it. We moved from shop to shop quite quickly as Elizabeth did not like being around people. If they started to crowd in we moved on to other shops, other streets, buying knick knacks and postcards, chocolate and lemonade. Our plan was to walk in the Blessed Sacrament procession in the afternoon, but I was totally unprepared for Elizabeth's reaction.

'I can't, Mam,' she whispered as we were stood queuing.

'Can't what?' I asked. Elizabeth took my arm and led me away.

'I can't face being with all these people.' There were hundreds milling towards the starting point and Elizabeth panicked. I had failed to realise how damaged she was and my heart was heavy; I was so disappointed.

'It's okay. We'll watch it from the balcony of the Basilica,' I said. We climbed up the long winding path to the top where we could look down and view the fantastic scene. The procession had started and a long, moving body of people was weaving its way right to the bottom end of the Domain to turn and come back down the opposite side towards the Basilica. People were crowding in on us trying to get a better view. Elizabeth became more and more anxious and then tugged at my sleeve.

'Come on, Mam. Let's go'.

We walked in silence back down the slope, out of the Domain, past all the shops and the open bars where people were enjoying a drink and gossip and arrived at our hotel. In our room, Elizabeth flung herself on to her bed and sobbed.

'What am I going to do? I can't go to the Grotto. I can't face all those people.' 'I'll think of something,' I said. What should I do? I knew no-one, but I had a programme of the Liverpool diocesan services. 'Look, Elizabeth. There's a reconciliation service on tonight. If we go to the church, I can find an English speaking priest and ask his help.'

Elizabeth rested and later in the evening we went back to the Domain, slipped into the church where the service had already started, and into a back seat. Everyone was encouraged to go for a blessing, a chat or absolution to one of the many priests now scattered round the church. We joined a queue. Looking around, I spotted a young priest and hoped we might get him as I thought he would be okay for Elizabeth, but when our turn came we found ourselves in front of an elderly man. How will he react to my plea?

'Hello. You're very welcome. Take a seat.' He had a lilting Irish accent.

'Father, we haven't come for the Sacrament. We're alone in Lourdes. I don't know anyone and my daughter's very ill. She wants to go to the Grotto but can't face the crowds. I don't know what to do...' My voiced tailed off and I started to cry. This lovely man never batted an eyelid.

'God love you,' he said. 'Wait at the back of church until I'm finished here. It'll be about 11.30pm, but just wait there till I come.'

The church was almost empty by the time our priest came.

'Hello, again. I'm Father Will', he said taking Elizabeth's arm.

'I'm Edna and this is Elizabeth.

'God love you,' he replied. 'Come.' Keeping close to Elizabeth, Father Will on one side and me on the other, we walked in the warm evening air towards the Grotto. He never questioned us. The river water was gently lapping its banks as we walked along. The crowds had disappeared. Father Will led us to an empty bench in front of the cave. There were a few pilgrims quietly praying in the shadows of flickering lights of the many candles burning. We said the rosary together. I gazed at the rusting crutches hanging on one side of the Grotto on the cliff side and Mary's statue nestling by a bush on the other. There was an atmosphere of tranquillity. I felt at peace.

Father Will stood up and whispered,

'Come, we'll go into the cave.' Elizabeth went close behind him and I followed her as we made our way into the small cave where we could see under some glass, water coming out of the earth. This was the source of the water piped to the taps for people to take home and to the rows of individual baths where pilgrims are immersed. We slowly walked round inside the cave touching the stones, shiny and smooth, having been touched by the many thousands of pilgrims who come year after year.

We made our way back to cross through the Domain, but the gates were closed. Father pleaded with the officials:

'It's my chest', he said, but to no avail; it was after midnight and the gates had been locked. We had to return take the pathway, which leads up the side of the hill over the Grotto. It was a steep climb. Father Will struggled; his steps became slower and slower.

'I'll have to stop,' he gasped, reaching for his inhaler.

'Don't let him die,' I prayed, not after all he has done for us. Father Will recovered enough to begin walking again and insisted on staying with us until we reached our hotel.

'Goodnight, God bless,' I said, 'and thank you.' Elizabeth voiced her thanks.

'God love you,' he replied and with that he turned and walked off down the street. It was after 1.00am.

'I'll have to stay in bed, Mam', Elizabeth said, as I was dressing next morning. She was exhausted from the long journey to Lourdes, the trauma of yesterday, and the very late hour we had gone to bed.

'That's all right. I'll see if I can bring you some breakfast,' I said. 'This will be fun,' I thought, as I went downstairs; it was over thirty years since I had studied the French language at school. Our table was tucked away in the corner of the dining room as Elizabeth did not feel able to socialise and I ate my breakfast before beckoning a waitress. *'Ma fille est très malade et elle est fatalité,'* I stuttered, not knowing if my words were correct and knowing my accent was atrocious. It got worse. *'S'il vous plais je prenne le pain à ma fille et le thé?'* The waitress watching my hands gesticulate that my daughter was asleep and listening to my feeble attempt at French, gazed at me.

'Non fatalité,' she said, shaking her head. *'Fatigué. Oui?'* I nodded. It sounded right. She added, 'okay.'

'Merci,' I replied, conscious of my shameful effort. She watched and was smiling as I put Elizabeth's breakfast on a plate and with this and a cup of tea returned to our room. It was later I learned *'fatalité'* translates 'fatality' whereas I meant tiredness.

Elizabeth remained upstairs all day and we talked, slept, wrote postcards, read and quietly sang the words of the hymn, 'Be not afraid' although we couldn't remember them all. It was 6.30pm when the internal telephone rang. We had a visitor down stairs. It could only be Father Will, I thought. We didn't know anyone else. I was right.

'I thought I'd come and see how you were doing,' he said. I was delighted to see him again and we had a chat. I told him about Elizabeth's illness.

'Your diocese has a Mass with anointing for the sick tomorrow, Father Will. May she have the Sacrament of the Sick please? I would very much like her to be anointed.'

'I'll have to get permission,' he replied. 'I'll meet you at 9.00am tomorrow, half an hour before Mass begins.'

'Okay, thanks,' I said, although I didn't understand what he meant about 'getting permission'. Elizabeth appeared and received a hug from Father Will.

'God love you,' he said on leaving.

Over our evening meal I told her about tomorrow. She was rested now and we went to the Domain to watch the torch light procession. It was a tremendous sight, a slow moving body of people holding candles that glowed ethereally inside the paper holders. Afterwards we had a drink sitting outside our hotel on our own, but happy to watch the world go by.

'I'm sorry, but Elizabeth can't be anointed at the Mass. She doesn't have a badge,' was Father Will's greeting the next day. I stared at him in disbelief. It was a beautiful sunny hot day and I had been so looking forward to this.

'What do you mean, she doesn't have a badge?' I asked. He explained that at the insistence of the authorities in Lourdes, the clergy of each pilgrimage anoint only their own sick people. Each sick person to be anointed has a badge showing their name and diocese to which they belong. This meant nothing to me. I was unaware of this sort of regulation.

'Father Will, 'I said, 'I'm asking for a Sacrament. Elizabeth has been at death's door. She is still very ill. She is under two consultants. No priest has been across our doorstep and you're telling me she can't be anointed because she doesn't have a badge! Christ wouldn't mind if she didn't have a badge.' I was almost hysterical. The pain of rejection was intense.

'I'm sorry. I'm sorry. I did try, but it's all organised beforehand. I'll do it myself. I have my oils with me. I hope I'm in order. We'll do it before Mass.' We went into the large church which was already filling with people. Elizabeth took one look and said, 'Let's go, Mam.'

I realised that she probably couldn't have managed the Mass anyway, but the damage was done. I was hurting terribly. Father Will took us to the adjoining small chapel where we sat down on a little wooden bench. There he administered the Sacrament, Elizabeth sitting between us, both her and me very emotional and weeping quietly. It was a beautiful short service, but I still felt we were a bit like lepers because of her mental illness. The stigma is strong. I had come all the way to Lourdes and still had to fight for her. I realised with hindsight that it was not the illness, but the red tape that was the cause, and, already feeling neglected by the Church, I took this as another downside. In fact, I was hurting so much that I was beginning to ask myself if my Church was the Church of Christ that I loved so much.

We thanked Father Will and walked out into the sunshine.

'You know Mam,' said Elizabeth, as we crossed the Domain and saw the young adults pushing the sick and elderly people, 'it's all right if you are old and sick, or if you have a physical illness or are disabled, but what about young people with an illness like mine? What about us?' I had no answer.

Nevertheless, we had a good day; more shopping and lots of cards to post. Later, when the Blessed Sacrament procession was taking place, we went by ourselves to the Grotto, for it was quiet then. Elizabeth, counting out her francs, bought a large candle and placed it in one of the numerous holders before lighting it. We also drank the fresh spring water from one of the many taps before sitting down in front of the cave to pray. I cried quietly, allowing the tears to run freely.

Later, when walking back to our hotel I spotted Father Will.

'Look,' I said to Elizabeth, 'there's Father Will.' We walked over to him and chatted. It was good to recognise one person. 'Father Will,' I said eventually, 'it's now Friday and I haven't been to Mass in Lourdes because Elizabeth can't face the crowds. Do you think we could have Mass somewhere for Elizabeth and me?' 'I'll see if I can get permission,' was his reply. Something snapped inside me. 'This bloody red tape,' I retorted.

'It's all right. I'll say it somewhere even if it's in your hotel room,' answered Father Will. 'I'll organise something for tomorrow.' I felt for Father Will. He wasn't a well man himself and it can't have been easy for him trying to fit Elizabeth and me into his already busy schedule.

After the evening meal, a nurse, a friend of Father Will's, came to the hotel to see how we were and had a drink with us, which I thought was very kind of her. Later that night, we lay in our beds singing again. Long after Elizabeth had fallen asleep, I tossed and turned unable to get the words spoken to me earlier out of my head:

'I'm sorry but she doesn't have a badge.' I sat up and hunted around until I found a piece of scrap paper. On it I poured out my feelings, my pain about the Church I love.

'I don't need a reply,' I wrote. 'I just need to tell someone.' I placed it in an envelope, sealed it and addressed it to a priest in England before falling into a troubled sleep.

It was a tiny chapel where we met Father Will for Mass at 3.30pm. He had brought Mick, a friend, with him.

'I hope this is worth it,' Elizabeth had said, as we slowly walked in the hot sun down the outside of the Domain to the chapel. During the Mass Father Will said special prayers for Elizabeth. He was 'Christ' for me. He didn't understand Elizabeth's illness, but he acknowledged it and responded. Later in the evening, after Elizabeth had settled for the night, I left our hotel and made my nightly trip to the shops for some chocolate for her, passing the crowds laughing, talking and singing. I felt quite alone. I recognised no-one and no-one recognised me.

The next day was another beautiful, hot summer day. I love the sun. Elizabeth and I went off on our own to make the Stations of the Cross. We had a long, steep climb ahead of us. All the figures are larger than life; huge bronze carvings set on the hillside at various intervals and depicting different stages in Christ's journey from being condemned to death, through his journey to Calvary, to being taken down from the Cross when dead. Other pilgrims in groups were also following the Way of the Cross. Elizabeth and I stayed together as Elizabeth didn't want to join a group, but I was more than happy that she had found enough energy to make the climb. Afterwards we made our way down another pathway, across the Domain, over the bridge, on to the grassy Prairie and walked along the riverside. The water was sparkling and glinting in the sun. We could see the Grotto on the far side, but here it was tranquil with no heaving crowds.

At 6.30pm, we were back in the tiny chapel as arranged, for Mass. Father Will had brought Mick with him again and also three nurses. I read from Scripture and Father Will gave a short homily on suffering with special reference to Elizabeth, and she had a personal mention in his prayers. We sang Elizabeth's favourite hymn, this time with hymn books so as to sing all verses. I felt enriched. We left the chapel and made our way back to our hotel, passing rows of shops full of people. Outside in the warm evening air, we enjoyed a drink and, although again on our own, we were content just to sit and mull over the day's events. I went out later for Elizabeth's chocolate and decided to risk delaying my return by sneaking down to the Grotto. I sat on a bench and meditated and silently prayed before hurrying back to Elizabeth.

The next day was a sad day for us as Father Will, being too sick for the long journey by coach, was flying home. He had invited us to their Diocesan leaving Mass, but when we arrived for it, Elizabeth felt unable to withstand the crowds. 'It's all right, Father Will,' I said. 'We'll stay in the little side chapel. We will be able to hear. Don't worry.' Father Will remembered us and at the distribution of Holy Communion, he left his bishop and brother priests and came across into the chapel to give us Holy Communion before returning to minister to the pilgrims. He was a good man. I don't know what Lourdes would have been like for us without him.

At night Elizabeth was restless and distressed because Father Will had gone. It was pouring down, but she wanted to return to the Grotto even though we were not suitably dressed. We could not sit down because all the benches were soaking. This would be our last time to gaze on the statue, the cave, the burning candles and meditate. Elizabeth bought a large candle to take with her as tomorrow we leave Lourdes for the long journey home.

* * *

Arriving back on our doorstep at 12.15pm on Wednesday, we had a quick lunch and then back to the Centre to keep our appointment. This was reality. I paid a brief visit to church in thanksgiving for our pilgrimage. My parish priest asked how it had gone and listened intently while I explained how difficult it had been for Elizabeth because of her illness. He was sympathetic.

'Go home, Edna and get some rest,' he said kindly. I was beginning to feel more supported by our priest and this brought me comfort. I sensed he was starting to grasp the seriousness of Elizabeth's illness. Two days later in church a nun told me that Sister Marie had been moved to the South of England. So she won't be coming again, I thought disappointedly. The nun also asked me about our trip to Lourdes. I tried to describe what happened, but could only gasp and stammer. I was hyperventilating.

'I'm... sorry,' I said, 'I... can't... talk.' The stressful week with Elizabeth had affected me. But was she any better?

6
WHAT ABOUT THE OTHERS?

Two weeks after our return from Lourdes, Ray, myself and Elizabeth went down to Reading for a few days to see Kath, Mike and our two grandchildren. We thought the trip might be good for Elizabeth, but as the week wore on, she had become more and more tired. She was becoming restless and argumentative. I recognised the signs of Elizabeth's behaviour and sensed a crisis of sorts looming. On the Friday afternoon, having just finished our midday meal, we had returned to the lounge when Elizabeth lashed out at me verbally and rushed from the room. Kath was aghast. She had not seen Elizabeth for some time and had very little notion of the reality of Elizabeth's illness.

'How can you let her speak to you like that, Mam?'

'She's ill,' I replied.

I went up stairs and found Elizabeth lying on the bed sobbing.

'Come on,' I said. 'We'll go home.'

'What about Stephanie?' she asked. We had planned to stay overnight at Stephanie's on our way home.

'I'll ring and explain.' I didn't feel Stephanie understood when I phoned, but I just wanted to get Elizabeth home; we would be near the Centre.

'We'll have to go home, Kath,' I said, 'Elizabeth isn't well.'

'What, right now?'

'I'm sorry, but yes,' and I hugged her. 'Thanks for everything, but I want to get Elizabeth home.'

It was good to be back home. I visited Paula the next evening, but not for long. The telephone rang.

'It's for you, Edna.' I took the phone.

'I'll have to go, Paula, Elizabeth is upset.' I went to bed at 1.00am. Elizabeth and I saw our doctor the next day. We had a long discussion about Elizabeth's future. 'As I see it,' the doctor said, 'you have three options, Elizabeth. You can take a year out to recuperate, which would mean repeating the school year; you can stay off for six months and rejoin your class and try and catch up the work; or you can return in September and keep going as best you can with time off when needed. Think it over.' What a dilemma.

We kept our appointment with Doctor Longman where Elizabeth, sitting very tensely, gave vent to her anger and frustration as she desperately wanted to be better. Doctor Longman suggested Elizabeth return as a day patient aware that she was far from well, but Elizabeth refused. She was adamant that she would not return to the Centre.

'It's okay,' I said. 'I'll look after her.' I went to Paula's that evening for a short while and cried. It was all becoming too much. Elizabeth spent days hiding in the corner of her bedroom wrapped up in her duvet. She wrote her poem expressing her isolation and emptiness.

Changes are showing and you feel all alone
the silence growing nowhere feels like home
Your life becomes night time No sign of morning
hands out to reach you but still you keep falling
The hours of thinking the hours of crying
So tired of living but scared of dying
You scream out longing but no-one hears you
they just go on living when your life is dying
This strange sensation drawing you away
making reality a stranger when you want it to stay

I knew more than anything else that Elizabeth needed to be loved through all this to get her better and I was there for her, but I felt the need for support for me. I called at the presbytery to ask our parish priest if he would come and see Elizabeth and pray for her. Although I didn't express my needs further, I wanted him to come and pray for us both. I needed his presence in our home to help me feel supported spiritually in my care for Elizabeth. I needed some inner strength. He looked at me compassionately.

'I know my limitations. I am good with little ones and relate well to adults, but I struggle with teenagers. I've had hardly any experience of mental illness and I don't know your daughter. I'm frightened I'd do more harm than good.' I admired his honesty and humility. I asked him if he could recommend anyone and he shook his head.

I wandered home feeling saddened. Something was wrong here. I was asking for help and my parish priest didn't know any priest he could recommend to visit our sick daughter, seemingly because of the nature of her illness. If this is the situation, I thought, then something needed to be done about it. This was my Church. I felt there was a gap which required addressing. Somebody should do something.

'What's the matter, Elizabeth?' I asked at breakfast on her second day of school. She explained how hard it was to walk into her classroom to the stares and comments of her peer group. Some had discovered where she had been hospitalised. She was apprehensive about the possible backlash.

'Well, there's just today to get through and then it's the weekend,' I said, trying to console her. This was a slow recovery, if it was a recovery. Elizabeth spent most of Saturday in bed exhausted. Monday evening she was again very tired and extremely upset. I sat with her for two hours. Was there no end to it?

Every morning I had to decide whether to encourage Elizabeth to go to school or allow her to stay at home. Was I indulging her? Was I making matters worse by insisting she went? Was it detrimental to her health? Tuesday morning I persuaded her to go and she went reluctantly, but later I received a phone call. She'd gone to her friend's at lunch time and could not face returning to school. My heart sank. Is this going to be routine? I had no car. I rang Ben.

'Can you do me a favour?' I asked, and explained my need. He went and brought Elizabeth home for me. She lay on the settee. I covered her with her duvet and she slept.

Elizabeth had days at school and 'duvet' or half 'duvet' days at home. We went to see Doctor Longman for a check-up, but it was really a question of keeping going. What could anyone do? Days ran into weeks. It didn't help to have comments from well-meaning friends such as:

'I think they go on too much about hormones these days.' I wondered if people believed my daughter was ill. We went to the hospital for Elizabeth's check-up appointment with the gynaecologist. The medication was to continue. And so my days went on not knowing if Elizabeth would get to school, and if she did, wondering how long before the inevitable phone call to which I would reply: 'Yes, I know, I have a sick daughter; I'll have her picked up.' I would ring round friends searching for someone with transport and beg a favour. I talked of nothing else.

Eventually a good friend of mine, Megan, offered to take Elizabeth to school in her car. She was very understanding of Elizabeth, having experienced something similar in her own youth. She knew the struggle Elizabeth was having, the turmoil she was going through.

'I see her hands.' Megan confided in me. 'She twines them round and round when in the car. It reminds me of myself years ago. That's what I did.' Apart from the times when Elizabeth was too ill to go to school, Megan continued to take her. But for this, I don't think Elizabeth would have been able to go most of the time. I will always be immensely grateful to Megan for this support.

I was now into the third year of my degree course and as usual searching for books to help with the specific modules. When on the phone to a priest to ask about a certain book, I unavoidably poured out my story. He sensed I needed help and he was right. He suggested I go down to the Pastoral Centre and speak with a Mrs Black.

'I'm sure she would listen to you,' he said. 'I think she would be good.' I thanked him and put the phone down. No way could I get on a bus and go to the Pastoral Centre, present myself to a stranger and announce that I needed to talk.

I was feeling isolated and let down by the Church. I felt traumatised by months of coping with the effects that Elizabeth's illness had had on her, my family and especially myself, and needed someone to show enough care and sympathy to actually come to me. I could no longer face a complete stranger and ask for help. I felt bruised and empty inside and I needed someone to pick me up from the side of the road as in the story of the Good Samaritan, but I felt everyone was walking by on the other side, hoping that someone else would be the Good Samaritan. Where was God in all of this? I rang the Youth Chaplain who answered from half way down the country on his mobile and I asked him about pastoral care for youngsters with mental illness. Was there any help? He did not know of any, but listened sympathetically.

I wrote to a priest whom I had met on one of my course residential weeks in Birmingham and told him about Elizabeth, her illness and suffering and how I struggled to find God in it all. In his reply dated 6 November 1992, he wrote me some comforting words and, with reference to Elizabeth, said that 'her sufferings are yours because suffering is the inevitable accompaniment of loving. What happens to her is felt by you.' How true, I thought. How understanding. Later in the month, I telephoned a priest to whom I expressed my concern about support in the area of mental illness and he advised me to ring the mental hospital chaplain, Father Joseph. I tried to call Father Joseph, but he wasn't in.

I decided that I wanted the bishop to know that I felt there was a gap in the Church's pastoral care where there is mental illness. He was in a position to change things, I thought, because he had overall charge of pastoral care in the diocese. The bishop of our diocese had retired and we had learned recently of his successor. In December, I telephoned a priest to ask for an appointment with the new bishop expected in January. When I explained the nature of my request, I was again directed to Father Joseph. I felt so alone. I could go away, I thought. I could live in a bed-sit and look after myself. I wouldn't have to go through any more of this. I was horrified. What was I thinking of? I have a husband and children. I couldn't believe I could actually contemplate moving out. I was just desperate.

There was little change in January. We struggled through good days and bad days with Elizabeth. And so it went on. On 16 January 1993, I went on a study day to a neighbouring parish and was introduced to Father Joseph. I had finally made contact with him and I briefly mentioned Elizabeth. Two days later, I wrote to him expressing my concern about what I felt was lack of support for people with mental illness, their carers and families. I felt there was a gap in the Church's pastoral care. I explained that I loved my Church and that no blame was being directed to any individual, but I felt this was an area of concern that the Church needed to address. I told him that I had spoken to least seven other priests and none had taken the initiative to help me apart from promise of prayer. I personally felt I needed more than prayer.

I knew in my heart that I was going to pursue this further because I realised that I couldn't possibly be the only one who had gone through so many months of anguish. I had been searching for eight months and was not satisfied with the Church support that I had received. There must be many more families with a member suffering a mental illness. Were they getting support?

The Church offers a lot of support in many areas of pastoral care. There are a wide variety of organisations and associations listed in the Diocesan Year Handbook, which is published annually. I searched through this and found one relating to mental illness: The Association for the Pastoral Care of the Mentally Ill. There was a contact telephone number at the York Pastoral Centre and an address in London. I did not telephone the Pastoral Centre because I felt unable to ring and leave a message with just anyone.

Eventually, on 23 January, 1993, I wrote to the Association in London and received a reply dated 1 February from the chair person, a member of the Anglican Church. He wrote that my letter 'raises many issues common to those engaged in caring for persons suffering from mental distress' and acknowledged that there are concerns about addressing spiritual needs where there is mental illness. He suggested that one possibility of support for carers is a form of self-help group and went on to say that 'there is only so much we can cope with. Direct involvement with the mystery of mental ill health is that extra that many prefer to avoid if we can.' He gave me a contact name at the York branch and mentioned that he thought our new bishop was the national patron. It was this last piece of information that finally helped me to decide to write to our bishop about my concerns regarding pastoral care for those suffering mental illness, their carers and families.

There were many people filling the benches as I walked into the cathedral on 11 February, a day designated by the Church as world day of prayer for sick people. After Mass, during which Lourdes was specifically referred to, people moved towards the hall for refreshments, while the new bishop was at the cathedral exit greeting those unable to stay. Father Joseph came to me and thanked me for my letter. We had a chat and he enquired after Elizabeth. He was very kind and I shed a few tears, as being reminded of Lourdes had left me feeling emotional and vulnerable. Standing by the bishop was another priest who beckoned me.

'This is Edna,' he said to the bishop as I approached.

The bishop took my hands.

'I don't mind you writing to me,' he said gently. This was in response to my apology in my letter for taking up his time. We talked about Elizabeth. I felt his compassion and concern. He promised to pray for Elizabeth and our family.

'But what about the others?' I asked him, thinking of my Mam and those like her. He answered by directing me to Father Joseph. I was elated that he had responded so promptly to my letter, written two days ago. He had authority as the bishop of our diocese. I felt that by directing me to Father Joseph, he had acknowledged the issue of pastoral care for people with mental illness, their families and carers.

Father Joseph responded to my plea and visited Elizabeth at home. I left them together with cups of coffee and they had a long chat. Elizabeth was an unhappy girl and hated school. Unkind messages were written on the blackboard and notes left in her books. Some thought she had been on drugs and others that she had had an abortion. I was pleased Father Joseph had been because I felt this showed care for Elizabeth and myself, although I'm not sure if Elizabeth felt this. Maybe it was to help me that I needed recognition of Elizabeth being treated by church personnel in the same way as other ill people.

I was struggling with my Mam too. Wednesday, Thursday and Friday she had rung very distressed. Her scruples and obsessiveness about cleanliness were intertwined with her spirituality, giving her undue anxiety.

'Don't tell me off, Ed,' she had said.

'I'm not Mam. I'm just trying to explain,' I replied. I always tried very patiently to help without any criticism or judgement when speaking to my Mam. She was quick to sense any change in my voice or in my response. More than anything she needed to be accepted and loved so as to be reassured that she was loveable.

'You know you always help me. I need you. Don't stop now. I can't go on like this,' she had continued, her voice trembling and almost breaking. I had tried desperately to console her. I was very concerned that she might 'break' and knew I needed to take some action. In the past I had offered to ring her doctor in order to get help, but she was always adamant that I tell no-one.

I happened to have an appointment with my own doctor the following Monday and told my Mam that I would ask his advice. Monday came. My doctor advised me to telephone my Mam's doctor, confidentially, which I did as soon as I arrived home even before taking off my anorak. I was frightened that once I thought about it I would convince myself that I was going against my better judgement. I was scared too as I knew I would have to tell my Mam what I'd done. Her doctor seemed rather disturbed at my account of my Mother's behaviour. I didn't tell him much as I felt I was already betraying my Mam by mentioning it at all, although I thought it essential he should know something of her illness. He promised to visit her.

Mam telephoned later that day. There was a long silence when I told her what I had done. 'You mean you spoke to my doctor about me?' she said slowly and emphatically. 'Mam, I had to. I'm so worried about you. I only told him a little. He's a Christian, Mam.' This was because she felt only a Christian would comprehend her strange ways especially from the spiritual perspective.

'I could have fallen out with you. You could have lost my love for ever. You took a great risk,' she replied.

'I know Mam, but I did it for you.' Tuesday she rang. This time I suggested she stop going to church on weekdays to ease her stress, as her rituals about cleanliness, especially with regard to the reception of Holy Communion and her obsessional prayer life, were approaching the bizarre. My word was not sufficient for her.

'I'll ask a priest, Mam, and get back to you,' I said. This she could cope with.

I rang Father Joseph. 'Hello, it's Edna. It's not about Elizabeth; it's about my Mam. You don't know about her,' I said and continued to explain. 'I just need you to back me up about her not going to church during the week.'

'Whatever you say, Edna. You tell her, but you shouldn't be dealing with this on your own. You have enough with your daughter.'

'Whether I should or not, Father, I do and have done for years. She won't let me tell anyone. My sisters know some of her problems, but when she is desperate, it is me she turns to.'

'I'll see your Mam,' he replied.'

'Will you?' I said with joy in my voice. I was so pleased.

'Yes,' he said. We arranged a date and time the following week. What a relief. What a blessing. How wonderful. Now I just had my Mam to tell.

I was also puzzled about Father Joseph's response. I had told seven priests about Elizabeth before the eighth one to be told actually visited her, and yet immediately I mention Mam, one offers to see her. Was it that Father Joseph felt he would be giving me support? Was it that Father Joseph was more aware after learning about me and Elizabeth that the sufferer needs help? Or the carer? Or that helping the sufferer is, in fact, helping the carer? Had I achieved this with my perseverance? Or was it about asking the right priest? Was there only one priest in the whole area who felt confident to offer this help? Is support limited to one priest in an area? Should not all priests be able to offer this kind of support? Was it that there were other priests able to, but not necessarily acknowledged or known to have the ability? Was it a question of communication? I had a lot of questions that needed answers.

On the afternoon of Tuesday 16 March, a member of my family coming through to shop in Middlesbrough brought my Mam at her request, 'to see our Ed,' as she had told them. She wasn't telling anyone her real reason. Mam and I spent two hours sitting in Father Joseph's front room while he listened patiently to her outpourings with some prompting from me. At times I held her hand as she was very nervous. It was painful for me. My Mam was severely tortured with this well-hidden illness. I knew in my own way I was almost as broken as she and Elizabeth. I had soaked up so much of their suffering.

Father Joseph ministered the Sacrament of the Sick to us both and I was deeply moved. At last my need was being recognised. No-one knows the suffering of people with these hidden illnesses. I had spent years listening to my Mam's cries for help and had carried my daughter through her illness this last year feeling more and more alone, while most others seemed oblivious. Carers, I felt, were the unseen partners. What could I do for them?

7
I BEGIN WRITING

This question of how to help others with mental illness, and their families, had been troubling me for some time. I had a great desire to do something, but what? Sitting in church alone, I had contemplated this issue. Over the last year I had spent many hours in here, alone, silently gazing at the crucifix and trying to make sense of my suffering. I could have filled buckets with my tears. Most of the time I had felt isolated and in my desolation had eventually placed myself mentally at the foot of the Cross—at Golgotha. I felt there was nowhere else to go and I believed Christ would understand. He had suffered intensely, emotionally and mentally in the Garden of Gethsemane. He had endured the physical pain of the scourging and the agony of his dying on the Cross at Calvary. It was his Resurrection that had made sense of all his suffering.

And so I thought, if God can make good of Jesus' suffering, then he can have mine too, to do with whatever. Maybe good could come out of my suffering in being used, somehow, to help others with mental illnesses, and their families. I explained my deliberations in prayer to Christ and asked for guidance.

It was after this particular time of prayer that I began writing about my experience of coping with a young daughter who had been suicidal. I explained how I felt that as a Church community we fall short of providing for the needs of the sufferers and their carers in what is a devastating experience for the family of a sufferer when a member develops a mental disorder. It was early in March that I had sent copies of this, my first article about mental illness and Church support, to a small number of priests.

Soon replies began dropping through my letter box. In a letter dated 15th March 1993, a priest stated: 'I think the points that you raise and, more importantly, that Elizabeth has raised about young people and mental illness are very valid and important, and it is only right that they are brought to the attention of the

Church. It is a good reminder for me to realise that this is a real gap and need in the ministry of the Church to young people.'

Another replied on the 17th March that, 'you are right about the difficulty of getting the churches involved with support for the mentally ill.' After receiving a further five replies in April, I felt encouraged to circulate more copies of my article. I distributed fifty during April, May and June to clergy, religious and laity around the country, including one to the editor of Priest & People.

I received further replies. One, dated 11th May, was from a priest, who wrote that, 'I think most of the clergy would feel so untrained to cope with this situation that, without being conscious of it, they run away from it. If I were a bishop I would want to be sure that the chaplains to the mental hospital were the good appointments in the diocese, and it can only be done by men who have a real sensitivity and insight into what happens to us... it must be with a heart that is totally open to the person suffering. It tears me to pieces... I don't feel, for the most part, that our clergy, or I, are trained or able to deal with it adequately, and when you speak of that real gap in our pastoral care you are touching a very important subject, but clergy training is for so many things, and this particular area is so readily left to the 'experts' that the spiritual help, which those suffering really need, is so often not there.'

I took my Mam three times in April to see Father Joseph. He was so kind to her, portraying a gentle 'Christ'. Mam explained her religious scruples, her obsessional prayer life and her many excessive rituals to him, while he patiently listened to her. He gave her advice on how to resist surrendering to her scruples and authoritatively curtailed her ritualistic prayers in order to improve the quality of her life. Previously the Sacrament of Reconciliation had been the only place where she had painfully confronted her illness. To go had been torment to her, whereas now she could open her heart in serenity and trust and also receive this healing Sacrament in an atmosphere of compassion and hope.

Elizabeth continued to be very erratic in her school attendance. In April Doctor Frost, the psychiatrist in place of Doctor Connolly, requested a family consultation. Jacqueline, aged twenty-three, was at the time living with us and Christopher, aged twenty-one, was home from university. They both went, together with Jonathan, Elizabeth, Ray and myself. Doctor Frost seemed to think that we were not functioning well as a family. As he had only met Elizabeth and I on three occasions, I was puzzled as to how he could make this sort of judgement so quickly. Admittedly there was a lot of tension and stress in the family, which under the circumstances of Elizabeth's illness, I would have thought was fairly normal.

The two older children were not sure why they had to be involved and we were all ill at ease when Doctor Frost joined us. Each person was asked to express their feelings about family relationships. Elizabeth released a lot of her anger and frustration at not being understood and supported as she would have liked by her family. She eventually started crying. I crumbled, listening to different members voicing their opinions quite forcefully about family life at present, a family which seemed torn to shreds and I likewise broke down. Ray seemed to take a battering of criticism and when at home later, was unable to speak for three hours. He sat on the settee wrapped up in his own pain and as he said later, feelings of guilt.

In May, Ray, Elizabeth and I had another traumatic session with Doctor Frost. His comments, his questioning and his insinuations about my relationship with Ray and mine with Elizabeth left me feeling I had been torn open inside. I do not know why, when we had already gone through a year of hell, that we had to be subjected to what seemed to me was an hour of interrogation. That evening I sat in Paula's house, smoking, drinking and crying. I was a wreck. It was this month that Stephanie's wedding took place with Elizabeth as chief bridesmaid, although there were times when I wondered if she would ever make it. My Mam didn't feel able to come and face the crowds.

Three times in May I joined Mam on the settee in Father Joseph's room, listening, holding her hand, reassuring her, hugging her and helping her when she struggled to verbalise a point. It saddened me to think that she had had to wait until her seventy-sixth year before receiving this pastoral care. I felt that if there had been more acceptance and understanding of mental illness in society, then Mam might have been able to ask for and receive this support much sooner.

Mam was extremely articulate, with a precision for exactness, but her scruples, as she called her obsessions, were sometimes of such a personal nature or appeared to be so nonsensical that she would turn to me at times and say: 'You know, Ed. You tell him.' Her prayers, 'ramblings' I called them, were obsessive and here the authority of the priest was crucial in helping her to cope as he could forbid or authorise as befitted the need and she would obey. This helped greatly in eliminating guilt feelings when she omitted to comply with her obsessions. She had a wonderful sense of humour and could laugh at her own idiosyncrasies. She wrote many poems. One I particularly treasure, 'Enough', she wrote when seventy-five years old after her second visit to a retreat house to which I had taken her for a few days for help and rest. Here she had confided something of her illness to two nuns and a priest, 'her friends'.

Dear Friends, once again we'll be saying goodbye,
A lump in the throat, p'raps a tear in the eye
And when you three reach the heavenly home
You'll wonder, 'Where's Muriel? Why hasn't she come?'
And you'll all wander out and stand at the gate,
And I'll come plodding—and quite a bit late.
And sheepishly smiling I'll say, 'Well, you know
I should have been here a long time ago.
But I met with a scruple, who stood in my way,
As he often has done on many a day.'
'You can't go up there,' he said with a grin.
Your hands aren't clean, and they won't let you in.
You can't go to Heaven, all dirty and rough.
So just get them washed!' But I shouted, 'Enough!
You've cost me a fortune in tablets of soap.
To tempt me again you just haven't a hope!'
And I gave him a kick. Where he's gone I don't know.
But I think it's the place where I hope he would go!
So now that he's gone, let us all go inside
To that wonderful place where no scruples abide.

In June and now over a year since Elizabeth took ill, my parish priest invited me to talk with him. I had given him a copy of my article and he was concerned about what he had read. We met a number of times. I explained why I felt there was a gap in the Church's pastoral ministry to people with mental illness and their carers and families. I spoke of Mam's silent suffering, the agony of the confessional box for her and the benefits she was now receiving from Father Joseph. I told him of my own feelings of isolation and neglect over Elizabeth. I reminded him of how, when I approached him the previous summer, he had felt unable to come to Elizabeth. He had felt so inadequate at that time.

'You know, Edna, I was trained forty years ago. I have had almost no experience in this area,' he said. He was gentle and compassionate. I wrote to him on 28th June 'to thank you for giving me your time and listening to me.' At last I had been able to release some of the hurt that I carried over Elizabeth and the feelings I had of rejection by the 'Church'. I felt, at last, that the 'Church' cared and that I was being given some understanding.

June was a good month. The editor of Priest & People wrote back in response to my writing earlier in the year with helpful advice on how to submit 'a brief article (700 words)' for possible publication in Priest & People. I was most encouraged by this and composed an article as suggested, which the editor acknowledged. On 27th June I had a letter published in The Universe entitled 'Help needed in time of trauma'. Part of it read:

'My own experience is that, as a church community, we fall short of providing for the needs of victims of mental illness and for their carers'. It ended with: *'Is the help you can offer in your community, spiritual and practical, known, so that carers know who to turn to?'* Publicity at last, I thought.

Christopher graduated and included Elizabeth in his invitations to the ceremony, which were restricted to three. Elizabeth had written to him many times pouring out her feelings and problems and Christopher was affirming of his 'little' sister, which helped her through her difficult times.

In July, Doctor Frost, having completed his six months as registrar, moved on and Elizabeth was again seeing Doctor Longman who allocated her a community psychiatric nurse, Ellen. Ellen became a great support to Elizabeth. She was a regular visitor to our home after her first introduction on 26th August. She and Elizabeth would spend time talking and Elizabeth grew to trust and confide in her. Elizabeth felt able to talk to Ellen about how her illness affected her family relationships, peer groups and friendships. Ellen always invited me at the end of their chat to either inform me of any decisions affecting Elizabeth or to ask if I had any concerns. On one of these occasions we discussed the possibility of Ellen visiting Elizabeth's school to explain the seriousness of her illness, the reason for her many absences and outbursts of tears while there. Ellen agreed to this and I was pleased. It was a positive step. September continued with Elizabeth intermittently attending school and the Centre, as well as seeing our own doctor who had always given us excellent support.

It was about this time that, when out shopping one day, I met the daughter of a neighbour who stopped to ask after Elizabeth.

'You know, Edna,' she said, 'there was no help twenty years ago when I was ill like your daughter. There was only my Mam. She got me through.' So I made myself a promise that that statement would not be repeated in another twenty years by my daughter. Shortly after this encounter, I told a visiting priest outside our church that I felt there was a gap in the Church's ministry to people suffering mental illness, their carers and families.

'Well, Edna,' he said, 'you're 'Church', you know.'

'Yes, Father, I do know and I'm going to do something about it,' I replied.

On a number of occasions, I had met a Catholic man whose daughter was suffering from manic depression. I had seen him in August when he told me he had begun attending a carers' support group at a local mental health day centre as he was desperate for help. I knew then that it was time for me to initiate some Church support. I, too, had been empty for so long and needed spiritual nourishment. And so I began my mission. I contacted Father Joseph and explained how I felt the time had come to call together a few interested people with the intention of supporting each other through Scripture, prayer and sharing. We agreed a time, date and venue and I said I would invite a very small number of people whom I knew were caring for someone with mental illness or had some interest in this field.

In a letter to me from our bishop dated 27th September, he wrote that: 'I am sure that beginning in small ways like this is the best way forward in a vital area of our pastoral ministry to each other. You have my prayers and best wishes that it continues to grow and flourish.' The small group of people I had contacted met as planned, but I found this first meeting difficult. One person chose to question another who was struggling to share her concerns. He continued by telling her that she shouldn't feel as she did and even gave her advice on what she should do about her situation. She hadn't asked for advice and I felt she wanted to be listened to. The atmosphere was uncomfortable. This was not a good beginning. We planned another meeting in five weeks time, but I came away feeling inadequate, that somehow I had failed. I decided to seek counsel.

I had been given the name of a nun, Sister Patricia, whom, I was told, was highly qualified in education, psychology and counselling. When I telephoned her and explained my dilemma, she said she would come to visit me and discuss the matter. On the 6th October, sitting in our dining room, Sister Patricia said to me, 'Edna, you can't give to anyone until you get some help yourself. You are so full of pain.'

'I know I need help,' I replied. 'That's why I have initiated this little support group and we have Scripture so that I can somehow find Christ in all of this. I don't want other families to suffer as we have. I want, somehow, to show that the Church visibly cares, that there is something on offer.'

Within fifteen minutes of our meeting, I was crying. Sister Patricia listened to me and recognised my pain and my emptiness. She came every week for eight weeks and I slowly released my story. I poured out my anguish; my feelings of rejection and isolation, of lack of understanding and Church support; my spiritual emptiness; my fragmented relationships with Ray, with my children; and of feeling overburdened by being everything to Elizabeth, her emotional, physical and mental support. I was a broken carer. It took more than half the sessions before this kindly nun was able to say:

'You've finally stopped crying, Edna.' It had been painful and there was more to come.

My husband was beginning to feel left out and thought we ought to be having counselling together. He was under the impression that I was talking about him. 'It's me I talk about and my feelings. You can join me if you wish,' but he declined.

'I don't want to talk to a nun or a priest.' he said.

'Okay, then, we'll ring up Marriage Care,' I replied. I was glad he had come to this decision. It was 8th December when

Sister Patricia made her eighth visit to me. I told her that Ray and I were going to go for counselling together.

'That's great news, Edna,' she said 'but I won't be coming again. It wouldn't be right for you to be seeing two counsellors.' The same evening Ray and I began the first of twelve counselling sessions and it was painfully hard. Over time, some cracks in our relationship began to mend, but I realised it was going to take much longer than twelve weeks to repair the damage.

Meanwhile, our little support group continued to meet infrequently and numbers varied from three to eight. I used to encounter a carer in the street when out shopping who always asked after Elizabeth and was totally understanding. She said that she knew something was wrong with me by my facial expression. Often we found ourselves standing on the pavement, oblivious to others, as we shared our worries. Her husband had had a heart attack some years ago and she said that the support had been great when it happened. She told me that when he later suffered a nervous breakdown, 'There wasn't any help, Edna. I just had to get on with it.' He was still enduring a mental illness and she began attending our support meeting, which we initially named 'Families under Stress', as I was so reluctant to use the words 'mental illness,' conscious of the stigma. We were now approaching 1994 which turned out to be another eventful year.

8
THE VOICE OF A CARER

The first major event in 1994 was that Doctor Longman discharged Elizabeth from the Centre. This was great news for us. In February, Elizabeth and I walked through its doors for the last time.

'Just think, Elizabeth,' I said, 'we don't have to come back again. We can put all this behind us.' I felt light-headed and full of hope. 'And you'll still have Ellen to support you.' Ray and I had had our final counselling two days previously. Two years of struggle, but now I felt buoyant until, when out shopping one day, I met a parishioner, a elderly lady whom I saw regularly at Mass.

And how's Elizabeth doing?' she enquired. My reply was positive: 'struggling but we're getting there.'

'I'm so glad,' she said. 'I have just being saying to someone that it was such a pity about Edna's daughter being on drugs and how much I hoped she would get off them altogether.' I stared at her.

'Drugs?,' I questioned. 'What do you mean, drugs?' She looked embarrassed. 'Well she was on drugs wasn't she? That's what I was told.' I could feel the anger rising inside me.

'Whoever told you that, you go back and tell them my daughter is not on drugs. She's been very ill and is getting better, but she is not on drugs.' The lady was apologetic. I walked home. I just could not believe it. I knew my doctor had warned me that people would look for reasons, would point fingers.

'They don't do that with other sorts of illness, Edna, but with this kind, they'll be looking at your family, at your school, trying to find a reason. You'll just have to put up with it.' I was still angry. It's enough going through what we'd experienced without this sort of speculation. And we weren't through it yet.

Elizabeth made nine days at school in March out of a possible twenty-three. On two days she had made an effort to go, but had been brought home and the other twelve days she had felt unable to attend. She hated school. It had become an ordeal for her. In order to avoid meeting anyone, she would not go to the toilets at break time and ate her sandwiches alone in a music practice room at lunch time. She would not come down to the entrance hall when I went to pick her up until all other pupils had dispersed. She was very, very unhappy. Most of her peer group did not understand the nature of her illness. I wondered if there were other families with children suffering like Elizabeth and made enquiries about the support group at the mental health day centre and the opportunities to meet other carers.

It was in April that I managed to make my way to the venue where the meeting was held. I sat down in a comfortable chair while a lady was speaking of her latest experience with her son, who had schizophrenia. Carers, desperate to meet others with whom they could identify, had initiated this support group. I listened for an hour before someone invited me to speak.

'My daughter became ill at thirteen and was on a twenty-four hour suicide watch,' I told them and briefly explained the trauma of the early weeks, the build up of feelings of isolation and the need to meet someone who had experienced this and come through it. No-one had met a carer of someone suffering a mental illness at such a young age.

'It doesn't sound as if things have changed much since our son was at the Centre. He's an outpatient at the main mental hospital now,' voiced one carer.

'We've all been there,' said another. 'I mean about you crying and walking home. I've walked the streets in tears many times not knowing who to turn to. This group's been a lifeline for me.'

'Do you remember when I bumped into you at the library and asked after your son and you told me and I was so pleased because I knew you'd understand about my troubles?' said another. And so it went on.

Some of their stories were horrendous. I considered myself lucky in that our situation was more bearable now. I attended regularly even though I was quite disturbed by hearing of the traumas and suffering in other peoples' lives. Sometimes speakers were invited. We were informed about benefits. I had given up part-time work to look after Elizabeth and was unaware that I could have applied for financial support when caring for her full-time. I was given this information at one of the meetings, but it was too late for me to benefit from it as Elizabeth had returned to school.

Elizabeth was due to sit her GCSE exams in May and one of the deputy heads had suggested that she might like to take them in a room separate from the other candidates in the main hall. This seemed a good suggestion as neither Elizabeth or I knew how she might react under so much stress. At times Elizabeth was joined by another pupil who was also ill. The build-up to the exams was horrific. We seemed to be forever at the doctor's surgery with emergency appointments as Elizabeth was constantly succumbing to infections. Our doctor and his partners were patient and obliging. The weeks of exam time were a nightmare for me. I was backwards and forwards to school as well as to the doctor's surgery. I sat with Elizabeth in the evenings and we had broken nights with her coming into my bedroom and sleeping with me. I gave her much needed 'tender loving care' on the days when she was not taking exams and encouraged and reassured her on exam days. At last they came to an end. Elizabeth walked out of school for the last time on 24th June, the day after her sixteenth birthday. We had made it through two years of struggle.

In August the results were out. 'I've passed, I've passed', Elizabeth called as she approached the car. We hugged and tears of joy trickled down my cheeks.

'Oh, Elizabeth,' was all I could whisper. She had achieved six B grades and three C grades. 'And you have those for the rest of your life and no-one can take them from you,' I told her. On Sunday the balloon burst. A group of us were discussing exam results outside church and sharing information on pupils' achievements. A lady stated how pleased she was to hear of Elizabeth's results and added, 'Now she'll realise how stupid she's been.' I walked away. If only people realised the effort it had taken instead of implying that her illness was a put-up job. Why couldn't they believe me? But other good things had been happening over the last months. My article submitted to *Priest & People* had finally been published and there was positive response.

It had been one morning in March that I watched the postman pass by our window and heard the letter box close as the post fell on to the doormat with a thud. I picked up a package and opened it. Out fell two copies of *Priest & People* and there inside was my one page article. It had been titled, *The Voice of a Carer*. I was elated. Now there would be a response I thought. A few weeks later I was kneeling in church praying to God in something like these words. 'It's a year since I started writing. I've finally had an article published. Nothing seems to be happening and I don't know what to do. If you want me to continue, you'll have to show me how.' I was feeling disillusioned.

I wandered home and into the kitchen to make a cup of tea when the telephone rang. 'Yes, I'm Edna Hunneysett.' A Catholic lay woman chaplain to a mental hospital introduced herself and told me that she and a Dominican priest had been to see their bishop about my published article. He had booked the meeting room at Newcastle Cathedral for the following to be addressed:

> *'Concern has been expressed due to the closing of mental hospitals over how we can best support carers of people with mental illness as they return to the community; to explore the need for spiritual support for carers, families and friends of people with mental illness; and to prepare our community for the discharging of mentally ill patients to their families and community living,'*

I was being invited to speak at this Open Meeting, alongside other carers. My response was, 'That's wonderful. Of course I will. About how long would you like me to speak?' The chaplain gave me more details before we concluded the conversation. I put the phone down.

I was ecstatic. I wanted to jump up and down and sing. I felt guilty about my lack of trust in God because He'd been busy all the time. I received a copy of the advertising poster, and had many photocopied and distributed them to churches, hospitals, schools and pastoral centres. And so it was that one Thursday evening in May, I was sitting in a chair drinking a cup of tea checking through my notes while watching people arrive. We were in a meeting room and all my thoughts were focussed on the fact that I was going to stand up and speak in front of this crowd of sixty people.

I was soberly dressed because earlier in the day I had been to my twenty-five year old nephew's funeral. His car had been swept off a ford into a swollen river on the Sunday evening and his body recovered by police frogmen on the Monday night. Jacqueline had announced her engagement on that Monday and we had gone to have a drink with her and Dave to celebrate. It was after returning home that I had received my sister's telephone call. I sat on the stairs and rocked and moaned not wanting to accept this tragedy. Ray and I were his godparents. The funeral had taken place in a small village on the Yorkshire moors attended by many relatives. Christopher was affected badly as he was close in age to this nephew. I came back to Middlesbrough but with no time to change before being picked up by Paula and Margaret who were accompanying me to Newcastle.

'I hope that the experience I share with you tonight will help you understand a little more why I feel there is a need for spiritual and pastoral support for carers and families of those with mental illness.' These were my opening words to this crowd of people sitting listening attentively. And I ended with *'I think about Christ on the cross saying 'I am thirsty* (Jn.19.28). *When he preached about the Day of Judgement, he speaks of love shown in action* (Mt.25.33-45). *As a carer I needed to experience God's love in action. I was thirsty. I needed a cup of water.'* I stepped down from the platform and returned to my seat, my legs trembling. After another three carers shared their stories, my friend, Margaret, stood up.

'It's like hearing about another world,' she said, *'a world we are unaware of; a world where people are living these experiences and no-one knows.'* Her voice began to tremble and she sat down. She told us afterwards that she had been very moved by the personal stories. She had found them mind-blowing. Eventually the meeting was drawn to a close. We were told that the bishop was to be given feedback. Those who wished to be involved in analysing the content of the meeting and plan a way forward were invited to leave their names and addresses.

In July, it was Middlesbrough's turn to have an Open Meeting which had been advertised extensively. I was standing inside St Thomas More's church hall greeting people as they entered and it was good to see representatives from social services, the voluntary sector and members of other church denominations present. Our bishop had already written to me on 7th July congratulating me on 'the initiative you are taking at St Thomas More on 21st July... please convey my very deep interest in this initiative to all who are there.' He made a brief appearance at the beginning to emphasise his concern for this very special group of people, before leaving to attend two scheduled meetings.

An overview of the meeting was reported in the *Catholic Voice* entitled 'New venture for carers'. Details of the three distinct phases of the meeting were described:

1. A selection of anecdotes from the carers of people with mental illness;
2. Some input from agencies/support groups for carers;
3. An analysis of society's attitudes: carers needs: the Church's role.

Eight points for action were communicated:

- i Networking between parishes to help carers realise they are not alone. (The feeling of isolation had been clearly expressed by carers);
- ii) The development of a group of carers of people with mental illness;
- iii) The necessity to look at the needs of children who have parents with mental illness;
- iv) The use of premises, on a regular basis, for meetings;
- v) Responsibility must be corporate/parish based, with named persons in each parish coming together to form a 'link group';
- vi) In trying to pinpoint what we mean by 'spiritual', it is important to take an holistic approach to include physical, practical and emotional support;
- vii) In-service training is necessary for our clergy; priests' training should include an understanding of mental illness and its effects on family and friends;
- viii) A very important issue was the need to raise awareness within parishes and try to overcome the stigma, which is still attached to mental illness.

We were informed that the recommendations would be considered further and then, hopefully, implemented where possible.

On a warm September Sunday afternoon, I found myself sitting in St Thomas More's church awaiting the start of the service specially for carers, this being an outcome of the Open Meeting. We were invited to come forward and light a candle for the person suffering a mental illness or for a family member who was ill.

'May I light two?' I asked as I reached the sanctuary. Father Joseph quietly replied, 'Yes.'

I lit my candles from the Paschal Candle, a sign of Resurrection and placed them in the tray of sand on the altar.

'For Elizabeth and my Mam,' I whispered, tears gently running down my cheeks and soaking into my collar. Everything was a blur as I returned to my seat. I sat down and my shoulders were heaving as I felt the well of emotion rise up in me. How I ached for healing for my Mam, with her torturous, hidden illness and for Elizabeth to have her life fully back and regain her self-worth. Those who wished walked down again to the sanctuary to be anointed. As I approached, I could hear the refrain of a hymn:

Lay your hands gently upon us...
You were sent to heal the broken hearted...
May we come to you through one another...
May we come to you seeking wholeness...
Lay your hands, gently lay your hands.

My Mam had been to see Father Joseph in July. She did not come quite as often now, depending on her need. When she was becoming stressed and giving in to her scruples and obsessions with her prayer life, Father Joseph would see her more often to help her back on to a firmer footing. To me he was a 'Christ-in-the-flesh' to Mam. She was coping well and still had me on the end of the telephone, but also received support from my brother, Tony. About a year into Elizabeth's illness, I had met up with Tony and unknown to Mam, had confided in him.

'Tony, you can be a real help to me, but you have to accept that Mam has an illness. She's not selfish or strange. It is a serious illness she has.' He listened and accepted what I told him. I didn't tell Mam, but from that day forward, as Mam's trust in Tony increased, she was able to pour out more and more of her troubles, and Tony grew in his understanding of Mam's illness and the torture she went through. He became a real confidant to her and his regular weekly visit, enabling her to pour out her struggles regarding her obsessions, was a blessing. She loved him.

Elizabeth was feeling much more confident and, although she still had a lot of buried anger, outwardly appeared to be coping with her life. Ellen came for the last time in September. She had been a tremendous support to Elizabeth.

'But you can contact me, Elizabeth. Don't forget. If you feel you need to see me, don't hesitate to ring,' and with these reassuring words, she made her goodbyes. We were starting anew. Elizabeth was looking forward to beginning at sixth form college where she was going to enrol to study A levels. It was a feeder college for many secondary schools. New surroundings. Different teachers. Many students who did not know her would be starting alongside some familiar faces. A fresh start and all the horror of the last two and a half years behind us, or so we thought.

9
THESE ARE PEOPLE

'Jen is here for you, Elizabeth,' I called.

'Just ask her to wait in the lounge. I'll be there in a minute,' Elizabeth replied. It was the first day of term at sixth form college and Elizabeth's friend had called for her so that they could walk to college together.

'Bye, Mam.'

'Have a good day,' I said and watched them chattering away as they walked down the road. It was all change in our family. Jonathan was leaving in October to take up his university place in Liverpool. Jacqueline had moved out and Christopher, having been working in Nottingham since graduating, had recently moved up to Newcastle to begin a new job.

Elizabeth made another step forward in October, although very hesitant at first: 'I daren't, Mam,' she said to me early one evening. 'I haven't the nerve.' She had been hovering over the telephone trying to pluck up courage to ring a local restaurant to see if they had any part-time vacancies for waitresses.

'Well you may not have the nerve at the moment, but you will have in half an hour,' I said encouragingly. She smiled.

'Go on,' I said, a little later. 'You can do it.' And she did. She was asked to go in for a trial on the following Saturday evening. She beamed.

'You see, you are able,' I said. I was delighted and proud of her, but when Saturday night arrived, she was very nervous.

'You'll be all right,' I kept saying, and she was. She was subsequently given one evening shift a week, which was shortly increased to two. This was a real confidence booster for Elizabeth.

And I felt a freedom I hadn't had in years. With Elizabeth's health much improved, I had been applying for jobs and in November was interviewed for a position as a Link worker at a local mental health day centre. I was familiar with this day centre as I was still attending the support meetings held there, as well as going to the Scripture-based meetings at St Thomas More's. Now I was going to work at the day centre.

'I'm a nutter,' was the opening statement by a dishevelled-looking, middle-aged man sitting opposite me. It was lunch time on my first day at work. I had been told about Craig—a highly intelligent person who had developed schizophrenia later in life. He had had to give up work and lived alone, struggling to keep himself clean and fed, with little motivation for either.

'You're not a nutter.' I insisted. 'You're a person with a serious illness that happens to be called schizophrenia. You didn't ask for it, but you got it. You suffer it, but you are not a nutter. I don't use that kind of language.' He looked at me in surprise. I wondered, 'is he treat like a person in society or is his self-esteem so damaged that he no longer feels he has dignity, but feels a freak or, as he said, a nutter?'

'You know,' I said later to another member of staff in the art room, 'each person in here is someone's mother, father, brother, sister, son or daughter.' It could be my mother or daughter, I thought. These are real people, but they didn't always feel as if the rest of the world saw them as such. They felt ashamed as in the case of Denise.

'I don't want people to know why I'm here,' she confided in me. 'I can tell you about it, but clients might think I'm stupid.' She was middle-aged, slightly built with black hair and a chirpy character, always having a laugh and joke. This was her cover-up. 'Do people think I want to be here? I wouldn't come if I was well.' Her illness was hidden and tortuous. Each day for her was a struggle to fight her inner fears and phobias, but she put on her 'mask'. Her only night out was once every eight weeks when she went to a prearranged rendezvous to meet with a number of other clients for a chat, a drink and smoke. And there was Ted, another client, who had his story to tell.

Ted was a thick set bloke with a shock of dark hair, balding at the front, which he often commented on in a jovial fashion. He was a jocular sort of person, always talking, giving his opinion and joining in the laughter. It was noticeable one morning when he seemed unusually subdued.

'And how are you today, Ted?' I asked over a coffee break.

'Today's the anniversary of when my Mam died. I still miss her even after all these years,' he replied.

'I'm sorry, Ted. Have you no relatives?'

'No, none. No brothers or sisters. I haven't anybody. My Mam looked after me. After she died I got so ill. I used to sit in the park a lot. Sunday was the worst day. There was nowhere to go. We even had our own bench, you know. You'd see the same people sitting there day after day. Eventually I got picked up by social services and ended up in the mental hospital. I was ill, you see.' Later that day I met up with Ted again.

'Where are you now Ted? Where do you live?'

'I'm in a hostel now with my own room. It's very nice. Others are there who have been in the hospital. The staff support us if we need help.'

'So how did you recover? What helped you this far?' Ted looked at me.

'I'll tell you,' he said. And he told me his story.

'There was this vicar from one of the estates, who used to come into the hospital, and he used to stop and chat to me. He said that when I got out, I could visit him. So I did. I started going to his church and eventually into the hall for coffee after the service. I only have one friend whom I visit once a week, so it was somewhere to go. Two or three of the women were real friendly to me and kind. I started helping with coffee mornings. Then I got invited on to the parish council. I joined a bible study group as well. Our vicar invites me to his Christmas dinner each year. So I always have some where to go on Christmas day. You know, Edna, I found Jesus again with going there. I'm happy now. We're going to have a new church built and I'm helping with the fund raising.' Ted had regained his dignity and self-respect because he had been accepted as he was. He had found Christ through the love and support of the vicar and some of the congregation. I was impressed and thanked Ted for sharing this with me.

'I don't mind,' he said. 'I don't care who knows.'

Over Christmas I had been thinking a lot about my Mam who lives alone. Later in the new year she would be eighty and I wanted her to have as much quality of life as possible in whatever years she had left. I felt that, as a family, we could perhaps give her a bit more support. She was lonely at times. She didn't encourage visitors because of her scruples over cleanliness. Maybe I should take the risk and enlighten my brothers and sisters about the seriousness of her illness. Some knew in various degrees of her obsessions, but others had no idea.

I telephoned around and we arranged to meet on Thursday, 5th January, at Grace's because she was central to us all. My youngest sister, Miriam, who does not drive and lives the furthest away decided not to come. When I phoned her she had said, 'Do you mean I don't do enough for Mam?'

'Not at all,' I had replied. Miriam phoned my Mam every Friday evening. She took her shopping in Scarborough when Mam requested and she was very patient with her when Mam confided in her as she often did, about her illness. Mam always told me how helpful and practical Miriam was with advice. I explained in more detail to Miriam.

'I think you're very brave, Ed, calling this meeting. I'll go along with whatever is decided.'

'Thanks, Miriam, I'll be in touch.'

'Do you think we should turn back, Jonathan?' I asked as I peered though the window straining to see the cat's eyes on the road. We were travelling over the moor road to Grace's farm house. Jonathan, home from university, wanted to spend a few days at my brother Mark's farm, with his cousin who was also home from university. My intention was to take him there first and then backtrack a few miles along the road to my sister's. The fog was dense. It rolled over us in thick clouds. I could not see the side of the road, only the catseyes, one vanishing as another came into view. It was as if the world we knew had disappeared and we were totally enshrouded driving along in a sea of fog. A haze of yellow slowly came into view. I peered through the glass—the yellow glow loomed larger. It was two lights—a vehicle. Brighter now and slowly passing us by. The lights had gone. The darkness descended.

Words came back to me. 'The light, Mam, the light, it's going. Mam, it's nearly out.' Words ringing in my ears. Was it like this in Elizabeth's black tunnel. It must have been terrifying. The hours I had spent by her bed. And then I shuddered. There was light for her at present. Would it go again? Would the darkness descend? Don't even think about it, I told myself. The mist suddenly cleared. We could see. Just as suddenly it was back, enveloping us with its swirling vapours. My clammy hands were sticking to the steering wheel, but I dare not stop. We would be hit from behind. I crawled along. A faint light—stronger—emerging before us and no sooner upon us than it disappeared into the blackness and we were alone again.

'What a night,' I exclaimed as I walked into Grace's house. I had finally reached Mark's farm, dropped Jonathan off and made my way back to my sister's. I was a little apprehensive at having to put forward my thoughts about Mam, although as a family we were very amiable towards one another. I went into the front room and greeted Amy. She was well aware of many of Mam's obsessions. She spring-cleaned for Mam every year and knew about all the tissues in Mam's bedroom, the countless tablets of soap and many toilet rolls stored.

Mam used to ring me when she returned from Miriam's upset because Amy had moved things. 'She'll have touched things, Ed,' she would say. 'I know she's wonderful in doing it but I don't know what to do.' She would be in such a state and I would have to calm her down and reassure her that there was no need to wash everything again.

'Well, Ed, what's this all about?' Mark asked when we had caught up with family news. I tried to explain and had sympathetic nods in agreement from some, but Mark looked across at me.

'It's just you, our Ed, you know. You're too soft with her. You have to handle her right and be straight with her.' Mark was very good to Mam and he and his wife were often inviting her to Sunday lunch, going to collect her and taking her home. She had told me about the many happy hours she had spent playing cards with his children. But Mark didn't agree with me about her having an illness. Others disagreed with his comments to me. Tony spoke in my defence. He knew.

In spite of this, it was a very amicable meeting and we all had our Mam's welfare at heart. As a family we are pretty bonded. One member suggested getting her to see a psychiatrist. 'You'll have to go through her doctors,' Amy said.

'I don't think she'll agree to that,' I replied. 'I put that notion to her some years ago and she was most unhappy at the idea.' We concluded that we would all telephone more frequently so that Mam would hear a comforting friendly voice each day. Grace already took Mam shopping and would do this more regularly giving Mam extra trips out. It was Jack, my youngest brother, whose comment some months later struck home.

'You know, Ed, I had no idea about our Mam's illness. I wish I'd known sooner. I would have helped her a lot more.' He'd grown very close to Mam. He took her to a whist drive every week at which she played excellently and often won prizes. He was totally understanding and sympathetic.

'I couldn't tell you, Jack. I felt disloyal as it was, talking about her to you all, but I really wanted you to understand Mam. She's not able to help how she is. It's an illness and she's tortured by it.' I was shortly able to reinforce this to my family.

'That must be an interesting article.' I looked up. It was my boss, the manager of the day centre, speaking to me, a week after our family meeting.

'Sorry,' I said, knowing I really should have been doing something else, 'but you're right. It actually is interesting. I was thinking of how much it relates to my Mam and maybe I should photocopy it and send each of my brothers and sisters a copy to help them understand.'

'Well do it then,' he replied.

'Thanks. I think I will,' I replied. I took the newspaper and placed it on the photocopier machine. I needed six copies. The article was about a woman with an obsessive compulsive disorder and of her suffering and struggle. I thought this would reinforce what I'd been trying to explain when we met at Grace's. 'Telephone, Edna, it's your daughter', called the secretary from her office as I was working the photocopier. 'You can take it on that phone,' she said, pointing to the one on the desk beside me. I picked up the receiver. 'Hello.'

'Hello, Mam, it's me, Elizabeth.' Her voice sounded weak.

I had become rather anxious lately about Elizabeth. She was into her second term at college, but it was her health that concerned me. There seemed to be some deterioration and her sleeping patterns were changing. She went to college reluctantly. She was irritable.

'Yes, love, what's the matter?' I asked.

'I just want to tell you that I've come home from college,' she said.

'Are you not feeling so well?' I asked.

'I don't know,' she answered softly. 'I don't know, I'm scared.'

'Well I'll see you shortly,' I stated. 'Take care.'

'I wonder if I might leave a little earlier today?' I asked of my boss. 'I'm concerned about my daughter.' He knew about the history of Elizabeth's illness and readily agreed. I had some notes to write up and I left after completing them. What would I find at home? Elizabeth was so pleased to see me.

'I was hoping you'd come soon,' she said. We sat down on the settee with a cup of tea.

'I'm worried about you, Elizabeth, you know.'

'I'll be all right, Mam. I'm just not so good today.' I left it at that but the anxiety did not leave me.

January had been a hectic month for us as we had put our house on the market. Now that all the children were leaving, I wanted a smaller one. Ours was large and old and had been great when all the children were at home, but now it was becoming like a mausoleum to me, an empty shell of what it had been. Stephanie had moved back temporarily and her husband was with his mother as they were house hunting in the area too. It was during this time that Elizabeth began having sleepless nights and coming into my bed, scared. She was struggling at college and was sometimes unable go. Her mood swings were more evident. The situation between her and her Dad wase volatile. Tension was rising.

'Elizabeth, you need help,' I said to her one evening in February. 'You must get help'. Her eyes filled up and I put my arm round her. I still wasn't admitting to myself that her illness was back. I struggled to go to work and worried all the time I was there. In what direction was all this going?

'You must ring Ellen, Elizabeth,' I said in desperation, one day early in March. I was sitting on her bed watching her weep. 'If you don't, I'm going to. You're ill.' 'I will, Mam,' she replied. The following day at work, the secretary called me. 'It's your daughter on the phone, Edna,' she said, putting her head round the door, where I was writing up notes in the office next to hers. She was quite familiar with Elizabeth's voice, having taken many calls lately.

'Thanks, I'll take it here,' I answered. 'Hello,' I said as cheerfully as I could.

'I'm going, Mam.'

'What do you mean, Elizabeth, you're going? Going where?'

'I'm going. I can't stand it any more. I'm going to go and get on a train and go to Kath's.'

'Elizabeth, you can't. You mustn't.'

'Mam, I'm just going, I'm going...' and her voice broke. The phone clicked and went dead. A member of staff was passing by.

'Are you all right, Edna?'

'It's my daughter. She's going to take off.' My boss had appeared.

'She's ill you know,' he stated. 'She should be in hospital. You'd better go and see to her. Go on. Off you go.' I could feel the tears welling up. 'Go on,' he urged again. I mumbled, 'thanks,' grabbed my coat and left. 'O God,' I uttered, 'let her still be at home.' She was. She fell into my arms.

'Oh, Elizabeth,' I said. 'What are we going to do? It's back, isn't it?' She nodded. We sat down on the bottom step of the stairs with our arms around each other, both crying.

'I didn't think it would come back, Mam,' she sobbed.

'Neither did I,' I replied. I couldn't believe it. I thought she was better and that we had put all this behind us. I was dreading what lay ahead. I didn't want it.

Elizabeth phoned Ellen. Over the next few days our worst fears were confirmed. Ellen contacted Doctor Longman and before the end of the month, Elizabeth was back at the mental hospital as a day patient. I wanted to scream. I wanted it all to go away. I didn't want the pain. I didn't want to watch her suffer. I didn't want to listen to her sobbing. I didn't want to hear her and Ray arguing. I didn't want to be torn apart again. I didn't want to sit with her after nightmares. I didn't want her crawling into my bed and Ray crawling out. And yet I did want to be there for her. I did want to share her pain so as to help her. I did want to hold her, to comfort her, to listen to her and to reassure her that no matter how bad things became that I would never leave her, never abandon her. I would always be there for her no matter what.

'You know, Mam, you have to live with Elizabeth to understand,' said Stephanie. 'I didn't understand the first time. I used to find it difficult when I came home. Having been here these last three months, I understand a lot more.' I hugged her.

'Thanks, Stephanie.' It helped me to have this acknowledgement. 'It's so hard,' I said. 'All the goings on with moving too, don't help.'

Stephanie and her husband had bought a house close by and were moving in at the end of March. We had promised our buyers we would be out by the end of March because they were already in rented housing having moved out to accommodate their purchasers. On the evening of the tenth day before we had to move out I went to answer the phone and when I put it down I walked into the lounge.

'We haven't got a house,' I announced and burst into tears. The sellers had changed their minds. I felt I couldn't take much more, but we urgently needed a house. It was a nightmare going through reams of 'houses for sale' sheets and doing the rounds each evening including knocking on doors without appointments. We were desperate. If we didn't find one quickly, all our furniture would have to go into store and where would our two cats go? The cattery could not take them as they did not have up-to-date injections.

We found a house and, miraculously, we were able to move in on the last day of March as planned, thanks to the speed at which the solicitors and building society personnel worked. They were brilliant. A new house. Would this be a new beginning? Would it help Elizabeth?

10
I WANT MY DISSERTATION TO BE ON MENTAL HEALTH AND CHURCH INVOLVEMENT

I had slept badly. It was very early one Sunday morning in June. I ventured downstairs for a cup of tea. I opened the kitchen door. I could see a paracetamol bottle standing on the table. As I walked slowly towards it, I saw a row of white tablets lined up in pairs. I picked up the bottle. It was empty. My heart sank. Elizabeth, I thought. How many had she taken? I stood frozen to the spot. I tried to think. What if she had? Oh, God. What a scene. And then I heard movement behind me. I turned and saw Elizabeth standing there.

'Oh, Elizabeth.'

'It's all right, Mam, I heard you go downstairs. It's okay. I was going to, but I stopped myself in time. I didn't take too many. But I don't want to go on living like this. I can't take it any more. I can't. But I don't want to die either. Help me, Mam,' she pleaded. I could only hold her.

Later in the day, the phone rang. 'Hello, Edna, it's Katie.' She always sounded so cheerful on the telephone. 'Edna, I wondered how Elizabeth is? I was going to have a word with her? Is she able to baby-sit?' Katie was a friend of many years standing. She had two children and when needing a babysitter would call on Elizabeth. Katie's daughter, Mary, now eleven, would have no other person to sit when her parents were out. She was delighted when Elizabeth went to their home. Katie admitted to not understanding Elizabeth's illness, but when needing a baby-sitter, rang and spoke to either myself or Elizabeth. Katie trusted my judgement implicitly as to whether or not Elizabeth was well enough. I would either pass the telephone to Elizabeth, or if she was ill I would ask her and she would tell me herself if she felt unable. There were times when I knew it was unnecessary to discuss it with her; she was just too ill. This was one of them.

'I'm sorry Katie; she's not well enough. She's quite poorly at present.' Katie accepted the situation graciously and sympathetically.

It was an important affirmation for Elizabeth that Katie and her husband, Patrick, totally accepted and trusted Elizabeth and treated her like any normal person who occasionally was too ill to be of help. Katie told me of an incident when comments had came back to her about Elizabeth and how she had tried to rectify damage that might be caused to Elizabeth. She wanted me to hear to make sure that she was explaining the facts correctly. Apparently, on one of the occasions when it had been arranged for Elizabeth to baby-sit, Katie's thirteen-year-old son, John, had been asked who their baby-sitter was, by a friend at school. When John told him, he had exclaimed, 'Elizabeth Hunneysett?'

'Yes,' John replied.

'Well,' retorted his friend, 'she shouldn't be baby-sitting; she's had a breakdown.' John had reported this conversation to his Mam and she had sat him down and explained the nature of Elizabeth's illness as best she could. Her son had replied: 'Is that what it is? Then she's okay to sit, isn't she?' And Katie had added, 'Now when you next see your friend, you tell him the facts.' What Katie had helped him to realise was that Elizabeth was quite able to baby-sit when well; that there was nothing sinister about her illness.

Katie also related how she had had unexpected confirmation of the degree of Elizabeth's illness at this time. Patrick had rung his friend to explain why he and Katie were not able to accept the invitation to his friend's house because they had no baby-sitter. His friend had offered his younger brother-in-law.

'Thanks, but our Mary will only have the one sitter and she's too ill at present, and Katie and I wouldn't be happy coming if Mary was anxious. Some other time we'll make it.'

Later in the week Patrick and his friend had been to a football match and on the way home, his friend had enquired about the baby-sitter. 'How's she doing? Is she better now?'

'No, ' replied Patrick, 'but she will get better. She's been ill like this before and she pulled through. She'll get there.' And he added, 'you might know her mother, Edna Hunneysett.' There was a silence. His friend finally spoke.

'Are you talking about Edna's daughter, Elizabeth?'

'Yes,' stated Patrick.

'You're right,' replied his friend. She's a very sick girl. I'm her doctor.' Patrick had immediately apologised.

'I had no idea. I would never have mentioned it if I'd known.' No more was said, but naturally Patrick had told his wife when he returned home. He had felt badly about it even though it was totally uncontrived.

'I had no idea that David was their Doctor,' he had said to Katie. When Katie repeated this to me, I was pleased in so far as that, although Katie and Patrick had always believed me, the truth had now been confirmed and I was also glad to have confirmation that my doctor grasped how ill Elizabeth was. It was very comforting to know this, as it sometimes worried me that I might merely be thought of as a neurotic mother.

The Saturday morning following Elizabeth's attempted overdose, I was sitting after Mass in church quietly weeping and Father Desmond came over to me. I told him through my tears of Elizabeth's illness. He was new to the parish and didn't know her.

'I'll come and see her,' he said.

'Thanks, Father,' I whispered. Later that morning he arrived at our house and Elizabeth and I sat with him in the kitchen. She looked pale and drawn with dark shadows under her eyes through lack of sleep. She told him how she felt. It was obvious that she was in a severe depression. He didn't know what to say, but I felt he showed compassion by coming and listening and I appreciated this.

Three days later, he found me again in church.

'I've thought about you and Elizabeth all weekend. I couldn't sleep because her face kept coming into my mind. I don't know how to help, Edna, but maybe a woman will be better than me for you. I asked a fellow priest who knows of a Catholic counsellor who would be more than happy to see you if you would like to talk with her.' He gave me a name and number. I thanked him for this information and contacted the lady in question who lived quite close by. Somehow it helped me to know that she was a trained counsellor and a Catholic. I went a number of times to see her. She was quite happy for me to go irregularly when I felt the need. It helped greatly to know that I could do this when desperate. I felt better for seeing her as she helped me lift my low self-esteem, this a side effect of the stress I was under.

It had been coming up to three months since we moved house when Elizabeth's threat of overdosing took place. It was now the middle of June. I continued to work and Elizabeth was still putting in a couple of nights at the restaurant. She had only been a day patient at the mental hospital for a week and could not see the point in going. So again she stayed at home. She rang me frequently at work and on occasions I left early to be with her. Ellen was visiting her regularly and we had appointments to keep with the consultant psychiatrist. We also saw our doctor for discussion on Elizabeth's progress. But Elizabeth was ill and desperately unhappy. She occupied herself on good days by decorating. She tormented Ray into helping to decorate her bedroom even though he was very tired and stressed out with his work. She was erratic in her behaviour and verbally very argumentative and negative about life. The attempted overdose was a cry for help.

But this time round, as well as having the counsellor to go to when desperate, I also had the support of the carers' group. On the last Thursday evening of the month, I drove over to St. Thomas More's church and went into the small hall. I sat down and looked at the lighted candle and the open bible which Sister Dierdre had placed on the table ready for us. She entered the hall.

'And how are things with you, Edna?' she asked.

'Not so good,' I replied.' She sat down beside me. Soon there were six seated in a semicircle with Father Joseph who had joined us. He welcomed everyone and briefly explained the format, the sharing of Scripture and whatever else people might like to say arising from this sharing. Often we tried to see it in the context of our present day circumstances. He emphasised the confidentiality, the listening and that no-one need feel under pressure to speak.

We are light-hearted at times and even have a laugh in spite of tears. Some individuals are too emotional even to contribute verbally, but somehow draw comfort and strength from the sharing. We know we are not alone in our pain. We understand one another and are no longer isolated. I feel supported in this atmosphere and receive consolation from the sharing and empathy. We hear of God's love for us, which we find through each other. Father Joseph draws the meeting to a close with a short prayer.

'Are you joining us for a drink afterwards?' I asked a carer. Some of us were retiring to the pub around the corner to continue our conversation. I come home refreshed and strengthened a little and more ready to face the difficult days ahead.

A week later I had spent a particularly stressful evening alone with Elizabeth. Her verbal anger had been fired at me incessantly like arrows piercing me. She had just turned seventeen and felt her life was going nowhere, that she didn't have a life. She only existed. Her peer group were coming to the end of their first year at college and here she was sitting around at home, sleeping or doing tapestry, but not living. She had managed with difficulty to work her weekly evening shift at the restaurant, but wondered if she would ever be doing more than waiting on tables and washing up. She had been told at secondary school before her illness set in, that she was potential university calibre.

'Elizabeth, I can't take any more. I don't know how to help you.' I was desperate and had soaked up all I could and still she continued to railroad me in her despair crying out from the depth of her black tunnel. How could I help her?

'Come with me,' I suddenly said. 'You can come with me and tell Him.' I had a key to the church.

'Where are we going, Mam?'

'Just come,' I said. 'Come on.' I locked the house and we got into the car. I drove to the church and parked. It was becoming dark even though still June because it was late evening. We walked to the side door and I put the key in the lock and turned it. The wooden door creaked as I pushed it open. We closed the door behind us. There was a tangible stillness in the empty church. Shadows flitted across the sanctuary, fashioned by the flickering glimmer of the tabernacle light. We crept forward and Elizabeth made to go into a bench.

'No,' I whispered. 'Go on to the sanctuary.' I took her arm and led her up the steps where she knelt down. 'Now tell Him,' I said. I moved to one side of the sanctuary to allow Elizabeth to have space to say what ever she wished.

She sobbed and pleaded. 'You know what it's like to feel rejected, to feel isolated. You know, like when you were in the garden of Gethsemane; you know, all the pain. Why me? What have I done to deserve this? Why are you putting me through this? Do you want to take me like you took our Charlie?' Her litany went on and on. I stayed at the side, sitting on a bench, listening, waiting. The reference to Charlie was profound. It was the nickname we had given the baby of my seventh pregnancy, the baby I miscarried three years before Elizabeth's birth, but all the children knew. I was stunned by how she expressed the depth of her feelings. It was so personal. I felt an intruder, witness to a person's spiritual life which belongs to God. We stayed an hour. Elizabeth relented. Her tears subsided. She stood up and turned to go. I genuflected and followed her to the door. Neither of us spoke. Shadows moved as the tabernacle light flickered in the dark. I locked the door behind us and drove home with a very subdued daughter beside me. We were silent, each lost in our own thoughts. Elizabeth had had no time for God since our trip to Lourdes, but somewhere there was mystery and I had had a glimpse of it.

It was a long slow ascent back to reality for Elizabeth, but advance she did, bit by bit in between sliding back a little and stopping, while still trying to see out at the top, to reach the world she wanted to be part of again.

'You know, Mam,' she explained one evening in August, 'it's like climbing up the sides of a really deep well. It's so hard and I slip and only a protruding ledge saves me from falling to the bottom. I have to rest and then begin climbing again.'

Meanwhile, I had decided to continue studying by doing a Masters degree. It was September 1995, and I was back at Maryvale in Birmingham. Five years ago I had sat here on my very first evening of my BA course and again, there were rows of us sitting opposite each other in the lecture room. I had been accepted on to the MA course and had come for the introductory residential weekend along with my friend, Rebecca, who was going to do the MEd course. We were all mature students, either doing the MA or the MEd and we each had to introduce ourselves and give our reasons for wanting to study our chosen course.

It was my turn to speak. I stood up and looked around the faces of students, lecturers and personnel of Maryvale. 'I am doing this MA because I want to do my dissertation on mental health and Church involvement. I'm not sure what perspective it will take, but that's the area. It's because our youngest daughter ended up in a mental hospital at thirteen years old and I don't believe the whole area of mental health and care in the community has been addressed by the Church. I think there is a gap and I want to do something about it.' I sat down. I'd said it.

As we filed out, a well-spoken lady came up to me and in a softly spoken voice said, 'You were very brave to stand up and say what you did. Your daughter's very lucky to have a mother like you. I have had a mental illness. I wish I'd had that kind of support and understanding.' I discovered later that this lady already had a doctorate. I pondered over her comments; why brave? But I knew the answer. It takes courage to publicise mental illness. My determination to do my chosen topic for my dissertation was strengthened.

11
TO CALL THEM THE 'MENTALLY ILL' IS LABELLING THEM

'And here we are again, Rebecca,' I said as the train pulled out of Darlington station. Rebecca and I were travelling to Birmingham for the residential weekend in March 1996. We were well into the first year of our degree courses and eager to know what was on the weekend's agenda.

'Do you know what this means, Rebecca?' I asked. 'Have you done research methods before?' I was sat by my bed reading through the weekend's programme. Rebecca said that she hadn't any idea about research methods. I was clueless, but we soon learned. The whole weekend was focussed on them, lecture after lecture, beginning with theoretical issues. It was a whole new vocabulary to me: data analysis, positivism, phenomenological approach, quantitative and qualitative processes, operationalism, and inductivism. My head was reeling. The fourth lecture was a workshop on questionnaires, their construction and pitfalls and the measures of variables. I was desperately trying to make notes and absorb the meaning of the information, as it was essential to understand it in order to be able to carry out the fieldwork necessary for my dissertation.

Rebecca and I took our seats on the train at Birmingham New Street Station for the journey back home.

'How are we going to do it?' I asked. We had been given two research method assignments to complete, working in pairs, to be returned by early May. One was a questionnaire design and the other a data analysis report. As Rebecca and I lived quite close to each other, we were able to spend many evenings together over the following weeks completing these assignments. I found this concentrated effort on top of continuing with my module assignments very arduous.

I was finding it more and more difficult to combine working full-time, with my studies, as well as running our home, being there for Ray and our eight adult children as and when needed.

Elizabeth having celebrated her eighteen birthday in June. Our third grandchild was due in October. Ray was finding his work increasingly stressful. My health was deteriorating and something had to give. It is almost as if when Elizabeth is on the way to recovery I begin to sink. In May on the day after I had spoken with my manager and explained that I was struggling with working full-time, I actually broke down in our doctor's surgery and realised how stressed I was. At the end of June, I resigned from my work at the mental health day centre.

It was now almost a year since Elizabeth's threatened overdose. She had continued throughout with her part-time job at the restaurant and was happy in a relationship with a young man, Kev, whom she had met some months ago, and who was very supportive. She also had the companionship and support of her long-term friend Lorna. Ellen had ceased coming in the January and Elizabeth had finally been discharged as an outpatient at the mental hospital in the February, when it had been decided that she was well enough to progress with the support of our doctor and no longer needed specialist help. She had recovered from her relapse and was slowly taking charge of her own life. It had been a long haul back. 'But you know, Mam,' she said, 'I won't be able to fight back a third time.' I did not anticipate a third time. I could not contemplate it.

Elizabeth decided that she really needed to study and obtain the qualifications necessary for regular employment. She wanted to be more independent financially and emotionally instead of, as she said, 'Being dependent on you and Kev for everything.' However, she needed much courage to overcome feelings of shame and the lack of confidence due to loss of self-esteem. She worried about people questioning her past, about what she had been doing. 'What can I say, Mam? How do I explain?' We had many discussions over this. Does she cover up? Does she tell the truth? How will people react if she says: 'Well, I've been in and out of a mental hospital, but I'm all right now.' Will she be believed? Will she ever work full-time? Was she employable?

'I'll have to do something with my life, Mam, but what?'

In September 1996, Elizabeth returned to college full-time to attend a one year intensive degree level course for a Private and Executive Secretary's Diploma. She chose this course because she had always enjoyed working with computers and organising, and she realised that every business needs a secretary.

'It will only be for one year, Mam.' she said. 'In fact, only nine months if you take out the holidays. I should be able to manage that.' Inside, Elizabeth was terrified and confided in me.

'I know it will be a hard struggle, Mam. What if it's too much pressure? I've tried college once and look what happened. What if I'm not accepted but rejected and isolated because I'm different like when I was at school? What if I fail? People will think I fail at everything.' But she went. Each morning of the first week, it was such an effort for her just to get out of bed and dress. I lent her my car as she had finally passed her driving test in July and this helped her travelling to college. There were days when she had no energy to walk. But she was pleased with herself.

As she explained to me, 'I am somebody now, Mam. I am achieving, doing something people will give me credit for. I never thought I would be anything more than a part-time waitress, not that waitressing isn't okay, but I wanted more out of life. You know, Mam, I always felt people looked down on me because I had an illness that affected me mentally, that I only worked part-time, that I saw a psychiatrist, that I was different and now I can be proud of myself, Mam.'

'And so you should be, Elizabeth. Your Dad and I are very proud of you too.' Ray and I were delighted for her, but would she last the course?

I had a wonderful experience in the October. I joined our diocese on a pilgrimage to the Holy Land and in doing so, went in an aircraft for the first time, in a jumbo jet at that. I was a bit scared but Sister Deirdre happened to be sitting next to me and held my hand reassuringly as we were airborne.

I will never forget the hills of Galilee. I think I could live there. I was fascinated by the sheep and goats. They do actually follow their shepherd, not, as in my experience as a farmer's daughter from the Yorkshire moors, where the shepherd and dogs manoeuvre the sheep. Among other delights was sitting in a boat on the Sea of Galilee and visiting the Western Wall in the old part of Jerusalem. It is known as the Wailing Wall but as our Jewish guide said, 'We have wailed enough. It is now called the Western Wall.' I went there a number of times walking through the narrow streets in the old part of Jerusalem and passing the armed guards. I found the Wall had mystery. It had an irresistible pull for me.

The Garden of Gethsemane was compelling, especially a tree the size of its girth the likes of which I had not seen before. To think it was there when Christ was alive and visited this garden, that I was gazing at the same tree as he had. I was overwhelmed. So much to see. Too many memories to relate, but I will not forget singing '*See amid the winter snow*' at a Mass we celebrated in Bethlehem in a small church, with the sun blazing down outside. It was very hot.

In the midst of all this, I waited anxiously each day for news of the birth of Stephanie's baby. The telephone call finally came and the message was left in my bedroom. A baby girl. I was overjoyed and told everyone I met. We celebrated the joy of the new arrival with wine at our evening meal in Jerusalem, and I bought a cuddly toy camel in Bethlehem for baby Heather. But the peace and joy of my pilgrimage were not to last for long.

When I returned home all was not well. For a time I kept my thoughts to myself, but one evening in November I said to Ray, 'She's struggling, isn't she?' with reference to Elizabeth. He nodded. I had to admit it and was crying inside. I didn't want it to happen. I didn't know if I could cope again. In late October, Elizabeth had started having days when she was very tired, not a normal tiredness, but the kind which signified the onset of her illness. She was becoming anxious and irritable, struggling with her class work and sleeping badly. All the dreaded signs were evident. She started having severe vomiting attacks which lasted days. She visited our doctor who explained that, when her body gets to the point where it can take no more, it reacts by rejecting what she puts into it. But Elizabeth wasn't ready to admit she was becoming ill again.

It was in December and after her fifth vomiting period that she broke down in tears and said to me, 'Mam, it's back. It's been coming back for a while and I'm scared. I can't take it again. I'm losing everything I've tried to make good in my life.' My heart bled for her. I was on the telephone the next day to the doctor's surgery for an emergency appointment. I accompanied Elizabeth at her request. Our doctor prescribed antidepressants to help Elizabeth keep on top of things.

'Have you informed college?' he asked. Elizabeth told him no. He suggested that I go to the college and explain Elizabeth's history of illness and ask for understanding and support. We arranged an appointment. 'I need to explain why Elizabeth has been absent a number of times. Our doctor has advised that we explain about her illness.' The tutor looked at me, waiting and when I finished giving a brief history of Elizabeth's illness, she looked shocked.

'We had noticed signs,' she said, 'but we thought she must be pregnant. I didn't think of anything like this.' She asked if she could inform Elizabeth's other tutors and added that she hoped Elizabeth would get better over the Christmas holidays. I suppose Elizabeth's symptoms are similar to early pregnancy: vomiting, tiredness and irritability and natural conclusions had been drawn, but Elizabeth was not pregnant. Her illness was invisible. Ray was also struggling with work and was even contemplating the possibility of finishing. He was very stressed. I was the go-between.

I was also learning a lot about mental illness. I had been feeling uneasy for months over the name I used to describe our support group because of using the label 'mentally ill'. I decided the name needed changing and I spent time with Father Joseph discussing this. Instead of *Family and Friends of the Mentally Ill,* we decided on *Friendship and Spiritual Support for Families and Carers of People with Mental Illness*. These sufferers are people and to call them the 'Mentally Ill' is labelling them and is taking away their personhood and dignity. It's like calling people with leprosy 'lepers' and that is totally unacceptable. I would go further and say that people should not be described as 'manics' or 'schizophrenics' because it dehumanises them. We have to give dignity back to these people.

The previous January, Ray had laminated almost two hundred notices advertising our support group, which Father Joseph and I had worded and I had distributed to churches, schools, hospitals and mental health establishments. In the following April, with support from our doctor, the notices had gone out to twenty-two general practices. Now these needed replacing and in January 1997, Ray laminated another two hundred, which I issued together with a paper signed by Father Joseph and myself asking that the new notice replace the original one. Although it was time consuming, I felt that it was all necessary in helping to raise awareness of the issues of mental illness and care in the community.

I was also in communication with the Anglican chaplain to the mental hospital who had discussed with me the idea of having book marks printed advertising our support group. She thought that they could be placed in the information packs that are received by people in hospital. She suggested that on one side we print details of our group; when it meets, at what time, the venue, my name, the church's name and our telephone numbers. On the other side she suggested having the chaplaincy's number at the mental hospital for those who might want support on a one-to-one basis. It seemed an excellent idea. I discussed the wording with Father Joseph and we decided to add a quote from Scripture:

> *'Come to me all you who labour and are overburdened and I will give you rest' (Mt.11.180).*

The Anglican chaplain had 1000 of these book marks printed and laminated. She kept 100 and I received delivery of the remainder in July 1997. I spent many weeks posting them to individuals, to clergy of many denominations and to personnel of mental health establishments and voluntary organisations.

Nineteen-ninety-seven was a busy time for me. In the January, Rebecca and I had been back to Birmingham for another residential weekend at Maryvale. What this time we had wondered? We had to submit a proposal for a dissertation by the end of February. We were discussing the weekend on the journey back home.

'I don't know how to format one,' said Rebecca. Neither did I, but I knew mine was going to be in the field of mental health. How to submit a proposal even with guidelines was, I knew, going to be a difficult task. In March we were at Maryvale again and our proposals had been dissected and constructively criticised. I struggled to convince my tutor how important to me was the concept of my proposal even though I'd made such a mess in its formatting. My tutor questioned my ability to be objective on a subject in which I was so emotionally involved. I became angry. I was in a vulnerable state because Elizabeth's health was deteriorating and my tears weren't far from the surface. It was a painful learning session, but I came home resolved to go forward with my chosen topic.

Elizabeth had picked up for a while because of her medication and had taken some exams, but her attendance at college was erratic. She was having periods of incessant crying and her 'duvet' days were increasing. I came home from Birmingham to signs of further disintegration of Elizabeth's health. As we moved in to April, Elizabeth's deterioration continued. She complained of aching all over. She was constantly drained of energy. She was having nightmares and coming into our bedroom at all hours of the night. As she wrote later, 'The light was gone and the tunnel was black. I'd hit the bottom of the pit.' I knew she was very ill again. All the signs were recognisable. I telephoned our doctor. 'Elizabeth is ill again.'

'How do you mean?' he questioned. I explained and the following day we were back in his surgery.

Elizabeth explained through her tears all that she was experiencing. Our doctor took hold of her hands and said, 'up to now, Elizabeth, I have always let you make your own decisions, but this time, as your doctor, I am making the decision. I'm withdrawing you from college as from this moment. You are not going back and you're not sitting your exams.' I was devastated for Elizabeth. It was only six weeks to the end of her course. She had come so far and it was all going to be taken from under her feet because of this wretched illness.

Elizabeth told me afterwards that at that point 'The tunnel walls were falling in around me. The well was filling up with water. I was drowning. I couldn't breathe.' She implored our doctor, 'only six more weeks' and begged him not to do it and in turn he was saying, 'please Elizabeth, let me help you.' She turned to me, her eyes pleading. 'What am I going to do?' she implored. I felt her pain. It hurt so much. Why did my daughter have to suffer like this.

Our doctor turned to me for support, but I didn't know which would affect Elizabeth most; six more weeks of struggle or having the prize within reach being snatched away. I couldn't make a decision on her life like this. Finally, the three of us compromised. Elizabeth would rest at home and attend college only if it was really important and she felt up to going. I would go with her to explain all this to her tutor and ask for work for her to do at home. She would still sit her exams.

We spoke to the deputy head of the department who was understanding and supportive. She commented that, 'It was a shame to lose such a good student.' I offered to liaise between college personnel and Elizabeth. But in the course of the next week not everyone was as understanding. One of Elizabeth's tutor's said to me when I went asking for work, 'If she's well enough to do it at home, I don't see why she can't do it at college.' This tutor obviously had no understanding of the effects of severe clinical depression. Elizabeth studied at home when able and couldn't guarantee to be at college at a certain time on a certain day. Within a week, we knew this system wasn't working.

Our doctor had been right. As Elizabeth said later, 'If I'd stayed in college, it would have been over much sooner than six weeks.' It's a frightening statement to hear from your own daughter. Her life came to a complete standstill. Elizabeth was in bed for a week in deep depression and spent hours crying. She had sacrificed her part-time work in the restaurant in March in order to give all her energies to her studies and now felt an utter failure. Was life worth living if it meant years of misery, never being able to finish what she started and always having her hopes and ambitions dashed? In June, Elizabeth would be celebrating her nineteenth birthday and had nothing, or so it appeared. The results of the exams, taken throughout her course, were coming in: passes with distinction, but the diploma had eluded her. I grieved for her loss and again was beside her as she struggled her way back out of the blackness with many 'duvet' days and tears. What of her future? And I needed to work at my dissertation.

Section II

Introduction

It was during the days following my return home from the weekend at Birmingham in March that my ideas about how to proceed with my dissertation coalesced. I was still smarting from an encounter with my tutor, when he had expressed his, understandably, deep concern that, because of my profound emotional involvement with my daughter, I would be unable to produce an academic and objective piece of work on my chosen topic. He also suggested that there must be some support from the Church locally, and insisted that I research this on my return home. His questioning of my ability challenged my inner self and, as a result, I was even more determined to continue with my chosen subject. It was one area that I earnestly wanted to research and the reason for doing my Masters degree. Without this focus, why would I put myself through such a rigorous timetable of study?

I had spoken with the Director of the Masters Degree courses and, although he was kind, helpful and courteous, I sensed that he, too, was concerned that I might lack the necessary objectivity to produce the standard of academic work required at this level. However, he encouraged me to continue. With hindsight, I realise that my tutor had done me a favour, as his advice to look at the local Church situation regarding support was very helpful when it came to gathering ideas about how to structure my research.

The prospect of producing the 20,000 word piece of work was a marathon task, on which I knew I would have to begin immediately. I still had a module assignment to complete and I was aware that examinations to be taken in July were looming on the horizon. We had been informed that our tutors wanted the final drafts of the dissertations to reach them before the end of the year. The dissertations had to be checked, and any necessary amendments and improvements made, in order to complete and bind them by the following March deadline. I had asked the Director if I could send a chapter at a time for him to look at, as I was so unsure of how to plan chapters and content. He agreed to this and so I planned to do this over the next months.

During these early days, the thought of the onerous task that lay ahead weighed heavily on me. In each chapter of this second part of my book, I detail a major part of the research that I was able to accomplish for my dissertation. It was necessarily limited due to the time factor and the stipulation of not more than 20,000 words.

I continue with my story of my personal journey with Elizabeth and my family, which is related at the beginnings and endings of each chapter.

12
REVIEW OF LITERATURE: CARERS AND CHURCH SUPPORT

I returned from Birmingham in March 1997, with ideas of what would be required for my dissertation. My friend, David, who had been my mentor throughout my MA degree, called within days of my return home. He had brought copies of articles on research into support groups relating to mental health. I told him of my tutor's concern about the choice of my subject.

'I'll help you, Edna,' he said. I explained that as well as researching existing literature already in print on support for carers, especially where there is mental illness, I would need to carry out some fieldwork. I planned to draw up a questionnaire and circulate it to the two support groups in which I participated, in order to discover what kind of support carers received, if it was adequate for their needs and, if not, what further support they would like.

I told David that my tutor had advised me to investigate what support was already available within the Church. In order to ascertain this, David suggested possible people to interview. 'You could ask a chaplain to a hospice, a general hospital chaplain and possibly a Catholic doctor', and, I added, 'I would need to interview a chaplain to a mental hospital'. 'The bishop would be another person because of being in overall charge of pastoral care,' continued David. Now I was feeling more confident.

'I have to submit the questionnaire and the set of questions for the interviews to my tutor for approval before using them, but I'd rather someone checked them first', I explained. 'Would you look at them, please?' 'Yes, I'll do that,' he replied. 'That isn't a problem.' He was so supportive and encouraging. I was already feeling so much better about my dissertation. 'I'll ask Father Joseph's help too. He's always taken an interest in my work,' I said.

'Is there anything else you have to do?' David asked. 'Well, I want to look at Church teaching to see what light it can throw on giving support in this area of need,' I responded.'You can count me out on that one, Edna. With your theology degree you shouldn't have a problem on that score.' I laughed. 'Okay, then but with you working in the medical profession, you might keep your eyes open for any relevant literature, please.'

'I'll do that, Edna,' David replied. 'I'll do a search for you when I have a minute.' 'There's no rush,' I answered. 'It'll take some time for me to draw up the questionnaires and interview questions. I'll also need to investigate to see if I can find any literature on carers and Church support. So I've got plenty to do as well as finishing my final module and studying for exams.' David left and I went to join Ray and Elizabeth in the lounge. I was beginning to feel more enthusiastic about my dissertation, and more confident that I would be able to produce a comprehensive piece of study, but there was a lot of work still to be done.

On the recommendation of my tutor, I had visited the librarian at Maryvale when I had been there in March. The tutor told me that the librarian would carry out a literature search for me with regard to carers and mental illness and Church support. I had been to her with this request and she said that she would post the information to me. Her letter dated 21st March 1997, reads:

> *'I've searched in The Catholic Periodical and Literature Index on CD ROM and ATLA Religion Database on CD ROM and found nothing on support for carers of people with mental illness. The only article about carers of people with mental illness found was, in fact, by you in Priest & People, 1994. The references I've found to caring for carers are enclosed.'*

This letter reinforced my belief that this was an area in the Church which had not been addressed because if it had, one would have expected to have found some writings on it. Although there were references to four articles or books, I was only able to locate three of them, but this was a start. I had in my possession two other relevant publications, one from the Southwark Anglican diocese and the other from the Hexham and Newcastle Catholic diocese. I managed to find three other resources with some reference to aspects of caring and Church support and after reading all of these, I wrote my reflections.

* * *

Concept of carers

One author, Chiu, points out that 'in this fragmented world carers include those who provide in society, spiritual, social, psychological, economic and health care and include lay people as well as the professionally trained.' He suggests that the psycho-spiritual components of a carer range from a very basic ideal of 'doing good unto others,' to a more sophisticated idea of 'doing the will of God' (Chiu, 1988). He believes that the psychologial needs of the carer do not surface in the development of this psycho-spiritual self-concept of service, but feels that it is not possible to separate spiritual life from a person's psychological life. My own experience of spiritual emptiness as a carer echoes this statement. He goes on to argue that it is important to acknowledge that there is need for an integrated understanding of what is a human being's psychological development, which is coupled with spiritual formation.

He states that a carer's desire is to achieve a better life for the one being cared for and tension is created by the inadequacy and hypocrisy of some service provision. While carers are obliged to adapt to limited resources, 'the psychological, spiritual, moral and ethical conflicts of caring continue to escalate' (Chiu, 1988). 'Carers who take their role seriously, will ponder on the doubtful efficacy of the caring activities', he feels, 'and they will also acknowledge the vast untapped reservoir of disadvantaged people in society'. I empathised with him on this point. He suggests that requirement of compromise constantly confronts carers and creates a powerful ongoing internal struggle, highlighting the need to somehow resolve this overwhelming dilemma.

Self-care of carers

Chiu continues by stating that it is a responsibility to God and to others for carers to undertake self-care because to neglect this is a disservice both to the ones cared for and to themselves and asks, 'when the spiritual and emotional energy of a carer is heavily drained... how can the carer be restored?' (Chiu, 1988). He agrees that if the love of Christ impels persons to become carers, then, logically, it would seem to suggest that God has to take responsibility for them. Oglesby (1984) believes it is in weakness that

God's resources are drawn on and strength gained, which otherwise would never have materialised. A good point I thought, in keeping with St Paul who states that 'it is when I am weak that I am strong' (2Co.12:10).

However, Chiu feels that, in reality, no amount of prayers being said can totally support a carer who is in danger of being fragmented and goes on to say that many tragic spiritual and psychological breakdowns have occurred in Christian carers down the centuries who have taken this as the only way of restoring their integrity. He agrees that faith in God underpins all carers' attempts at restoration, but God has established resources in this life to restore individuals and the Holy Spirit walks beside each person, but uses others to provide assistance when such support is required. Thus Chiu feels that restorative elements available in the world should be gratefully utilised when carers find themselves in need of care.

Oglesby states that the time may come when the emotional, psychological and spiritual energy of the carer is heavily drained, which results in a need for crisis intervention and that Jesus' response to a need was by becoming personally involved as demonstrated by the Good Samaritan parable (Lk.10.29:37). I found reading this incredible as it mirrored my own feelings as a carer, of dejection, of wanting a Good Samaritan to pick me up. The Jubilee Centre, Ledger and Burton-Jones all report that the Church, as the Body of Christ, has a unique role in supporting carers.

Carers' spiritual needs and Church support

Burton-Jones (1992: 61,65) says that 'caring generates intense spiritual yearnings to which the Church, in its pastoral care, and we as individuals, must address ourselves'. She continues by stating that carers may suffer a loneliness spilling into their inner lives, thus making them feel isolated from the Christian community, a point made by the Jubilee Centre and the Newcastle Diocesan Board. Where there is mental illness, the Southwark Diocesan Board (1994: 39 declares that the carer is aware of the reaction of the community in which they live and adds that 'fear, rejection and expressions of inadequacy and misunderstanding' may all be experienced by the carer and 'this will include their church'.

Burton-Jones adds that if it seems to carers that no-one can fully understand their inner troubles, then this can lead to a feeling of abandonment especially in a church, 'surrounded by people who seem not to have a clue what caring is all about'.

She goes on to observe that the danger can be that very little support is offered by the carer's church at a time when most needed. Moate and Enoch (1990) feel that there should be particular concern about the lack of support offered to carers of persons with mental illness from Christian churches and cite this as a challenge for the Church today. Apparently I am not alone in my misgivings. Jesus gives a wonderful example of acceptance, empathy and listening, Ledger (1992) declares, when he meets up with two distraught disciples on the road to Emmaus (Lk.24.15). She feels the greatest aspect of Jesus' ministry was his willingness to enter into the human situation and that there is a similar need to give time and energy to carers to allow them the freedom to express their feelings. This is what I needed to do and, eventually, was able to do through being counselled, being listened to by my parish priest and Father Joseph, and participation in the support groups.

Burton-Jones (1992: 60) believes that positive help comes from friends who are 'willing to stand alongside, to enter into the suffering'. The Bishop of Woolwich says that bearing 'some of that pain must be at the heart of the ministry of those who name Christ as their Lord and Saviour' (Southwark Diocesan Board, 1994: 2). Burton-Jones goes on to suggest that the unique spiritual help carers need, includes: being listened to, being prayed for, and being supported practically by enabling the carer to go to church while the sufferer is minded. This latter point was also cited by the Jubilee Centre (1990). She says it is necessary to welcome both carer and sufferer at church and to recognise their needs and contributions in the Church's worship and prayer life. This point is also made by the Newcastle Diocesan Board (1996). She advocates attitudes of acceptance and unconditional love, and possibly visits and offers of counselling. Both she and the Jubilee Centre suggest this may involve introducing Christian carers to one another or enabling a carer to make a retreat in order to recharge physical, spiritual and emotional batteries. Obviously, there are other carers who have experienced needs similar to my own.

Another suggestion of the Jubilee Centre and Burton-Jones is that of organising drop-in coffee mornings where carers can meet to help counteract feelings of isolation or, as she and the Newcastle Diocesan Board propose, that of setting up Bible study groups to help meet their pressing spiritual needs. All three suggest the possibility of facilitating self-help groups and of establishing Church-based support groups, which are lifelines to many and where carers can share without fear of misunderstanding. The local church could play a significant role in meeting needs not met by statutory bodies, such as use of their building as a day centre states the Jubilee Centre. Burton-Jones (1992: 141) feels that ideally, 'for Christians, the Church will be the strongest social group giving support' and the Southwark Diocesan Board suggests that the organising of specific projects to support carers ought to be considered. For me, all this highlights the importance of our support group being on offer if needed.

Church involvement in 'Care in the Community'

Burton-Jones suggests that the potential for churches in providing support to vulnerable people is at its greatest in this era and is a consequence of the Care in the Community Act of 1990. She feels that the Church, in fulfilling its mission to which it has been called, will need to assess to what extent it should become formally involved in providing care in the community, as does the Jubilee Centre, and perhaps consider the possibility of working in partnership with other concerned groups. Members could become actively involved in voluntary bodies. Ledger (1992: 74) says that it is in this way that the Christian Church, 'can help break down the social stigma attached to disability and mental illness and thus support carers'. I feel strongly that the social stigma is still prevalent and needs eradicating.

Ledger (1992: 145) concludes that were Jesus here today in person he would be aware of carers' deep emotional and spiritual needs. The Jubilee Centre states that it is through the healing message of Jesus that Christians can bring release to carers who are struggling in their spirits and Ledger says Jesus asks today that we be available 'to allow his Holy Spirit to bring love, comfort and support to the forgotten people—the carers'.

* * *

These examples from the literature reviewed reinforced much of what I felt as a carer, especially of caring for someone with mental illness. The authors relate the spiritual emptiness carers can feel, the importance of pastoral care, and how much carers need Church support. The reference to Church involvement and care in the community confirmed my belief that this needs addressing by the Church. My conviction that support for carers of those with mental illness is an area requiring more attention is affirmed by the comment that this lack of support should be a particular concern and challenge for the Church today. I was pleased I had finally written one of my chapters for my dissertation and was encouraged by the findings that affirmed my belief of the importance of having these issues raised. During the time I was writing the chapter on carers and Church support, I had been researching for literature about carers, and penning the questionnaire and interview questions. There were family events taking place too. Ray and I were adjusting to him being at home full-time after having taken voluntary redundancy at Easter. He needed space to unwind and reduce the tension built up as a result of stress. Our grandson Will, made his First Holy Communion in Reading in May and, as in the previous year for Jenny's, Ray and I went for the weekend, taking Elizabeth who was slowly recovering from her latest relapse, with us. She was reassessing her life and, in June, decided that she would try for part-time employment and, possibly in the Autumn, return to college to attain further qualifications. She applied for a position as a part-time clerical assistant, was short listed, interviewed and offered the post which she accepted. Her qualifications gained during the months at college were excellent and being appointed was a real boost to her confidence. In July, after she had commenced work, she joined Ray and I on a trip to Liverpool to celebrate Jonathan's graduation ceremony.

In the middle of all of this, I had taken the second year exams for my MA and, with reference to my dissertation, had been arranging interviews. When I rang to ask our bishop about an interview, he was sympathetic to my request and referred me to the Vicar General of the diocese who was most co-operative. I had also made contact by telephone with three local chaplains and a

Catholic doctor, and arranged times and venues for the forthcoming interviews. The design of the questionnaire and interview questions had been sanctioned by my tutor at Maryvale who had been most helpful. I posted the final copies to all prospective participants. My search for literature in the secular field was a continuing occupation with many telephone calls and letters. While waiting for questionnaires to be returned and responses to my quest for literature, I decided to see what Church teaching was relevant to carers and began my search of Church documents and literature. What would I discover?

13
TEACHING OF THE CHURCH: SUPPORTING PEOPLE IN NEED

I settled down one evening in August 1997, with the Bible and a number of Church documents. I knew that I must first look at the Scriptures to discover the basis of the Church's teaching on helping the poor, the sick and those in special need. To me, carers, especially of people with mental illness, are people who need special pastoral care and spiritual nourishment. In the bible there are incidents recorded of Jesus helping people who were suffering and the Church has always put special emphasis on the Gospel values of care for the sick, the suffering and people in need, thus following the example of Jesus.

As God had spoken through the prophets before Jesus came on earth, I turned briefly to the Old Testament for the source of God's teaching and followed this by looking at the New Testament before moving on to the Church Catechism. The Catechism of the Catholic Church is a statement of the Church's beliefs. I also looked at some of the Church's doctrinal documents, which specifically expound on its teaching of helping those in need.

* * *

Scripture

It is recorded in the Old Testament that the Israelites are instructed to love Yahweh, their God, with all their heart, soul and strength (Dt.6.5) and 'to love your neighbour as yourself' (Lev.19.18).

In the New Testament when the Pharisees ask Jesus which is the greatest commandment, Jesus quotes these two commandments and adds 'on these two commandments hang the whole Law, and the Prophets too' (Mt.22.40); and 'do this and life is yours' (Lk.10.28). This instruction is developed in John's Gospel, where Christ says that 'I give you a new commandment: love one another; you must love one another just as I have loved you' (Jn.13.34). This is further expounded by John (1Jn.4.17:21) and by Paul (Eph.5.2). Christ came to do his Father's will (Jn.4.34) and with Christ we must love God as our Father 'and love all men as our brethren, this being the sole sign of a true love of God' (Maertens, 1964 :248)

The second commandment is the sign of the first because without fraternal charity there is no love of God. God loved all and it is Christ who reveals this mystery of love by his death on the cross (1Jn.3.16). Jesus is the model to imitate as a suffering servant (Mt.20.26:28) and just as love summarised the Law, the parable of the Good Samaritan (Lk.10.25:37) is an explanation of the Law demonstrating this fraternal love. Charity in deeds is a sign of love for the Father (Ja.2.14:26) which includes sharing the joys and sorrows of one's neighbour and not judging (Ro.12.9:21). We must recognise and love Christ himself in all peoples because he identified himself with the suffering neighbour (Mt.25.31:46). His compassion was evident especially for sick people and their families (Mt.15.22:28; Lk.9.38:43) and his healing ministry was often of people with apparent mental illness (Mk.5.15).

Catechism of the Catholic Church

The teachings in Scripture have been passed down and developed in the tradition of the Church and in the Catechism (Part 3) is a section on Love for the Poor where Gospel values are expounded. It states that 'works of mercy are charitable actions by which we come to the aid of our neighbour in his spiritual and bodily necessities' (CCC 2447; Is.58.6:7; Heb.13.3), and spiritual works of mercy include consoling and comforting (CCC 2447). Human misery is depicted in various ways including unjust oppression and psychological illness and it elicited Christ's compassion, who identified himself with the least of his brethren. Those who are oppressed by poverty 'are the object of **a preferential love** on the part of the Church' (CCC 2448) and Jesus invites us to recognise his own presence in those in need (Mt.25.40; CCC 2449).

Sacred Congregation for Divine Worship: 'Hominum Dolores' Introduction to the Rite of Anointing and to the Pastoral Care of the Sick

This document sheds light on the meaning of human sickness in the mystery of salvation as Christ's words show that illness has a value for salvation of the world (HD 1). Christ knew human sorrow and 'still suffers and undergoes torments whenever we his followers suffer' (HD 2). Part of God's plan is that we should 'prudently seek the blessings of good health' (HD 3).

'It is the duty of all who have taken it on themselves to succour the sick to do whatever they deem necessary to help them both physically and spiritually' (HD 4). This fulfils Christ's command as it was Christ's intention 'that the whole person should be their concern and that they should offer both physical relief and spiritual comfort' (HD 4) because the concern he himself showed was for both the bodily and spiritual welfare of the sick (HD 5). 'If one member of Christ's body, the Church, suffers, all members suffer... consequently... works of charity and help given for the relief of human want should be held in high esteem' (HD 33).

Vatican II: 'Gaudium et Spes' Pastoral Constitution on the Church in the Modern World

This document shows solidarity of the Church with the whole human family. It teaches that a person should be considered, whole and entire, in 'body and soul, heart and conscience, mind and will' (GS 3) and that a human person is a social being who can only live and develop in relationship with others. The opening words remind that the joy and hope, the grief and anguish of people especially those afflicted in any way are the joy and hope, the grief and anguish of the followers of Christ. Just as Christ came to bear witness to the truth and to serve, so too, the Church is only interested in carrying out the work of Christ under the guidance of the Holy Spirit. In the document, it is taught that deep within a person's conscience is a law inscribed by God calling a person to love. A person's dignity lies in observing this law by which a person will be judged and this law is fulfilled by loving God and loving one's neighbour.

The Holy See: The International Year of Disabled Persons

In this document, the Church says that through the centuries, the community of Christ's disciples, in following his example, has 'caused to flourish works of extraordinary generosity... that bear witness... to the unrepeatable value of each individual human life' (p519). Persons handicapped in any way and their families belong to the whole human family, but may be in a minority. This may entail insufficient interest and added to that is 'the often spontaneous reaction of a community that rejects and psychologically represses that which does not fit into its habits' (p526). People do not want to face negative aspects of life, but this gives rise to exclusion and discrimination and, therefore, this tendency must be countered by education. People behave in a way that is truly human when they enter into a process 'of accepting even weakness, of solidarity and of sharing in others' sufferings' (p526). As witnesses to Christ, Christians must adopt his sentiments towards the suffering and stimulate this attitude in the world by example.

The Church teaches that, 'the quality of a society and a civilisation is measured by the respect shown to the weakest of its members' (p520). It is necessary to reflect on the distressing situation of the many people who undergo stress and shock that disturb their psychic and interior life and it is important that the health of the spirit is fostered so that a person is not damaged in his deeper needs.

It says that, 'spiritual ecology is needed as much as natural ecology' (p522). Those responsible for planning programmes in social care and integration of disabled people should make the family the starting point as families need to be given great understanding and sympathy so as to help prevent feelings of isolation and rejection. Heroic strength of mind is required by these families and the witness which these families give to the dignity and sacredness and values of the human person deserve open recognition and support by the whole community. Also professionals and volunteers who give themselves to the service of the disabled should 'learn to dialogue with the parents and families' (p526).

John Paul II: 'Familiaris Consortio' The Christian Family in the Modern World: Vatican II: 'Lumen Gentium' Dogmatic Constitution on the Church: Vatican II: 'Apostolicam Actuositatem' Decree on the Apostolate of lay People

The Second Vatican Council identified in Christ's attitude towards the suffering the essential core of the apostolate of lay people, in that Christ made love of neighbour his personal commandment and 'charity the distinguishing mark of his disciples' (p527). Christians need to stand alongside organisations to foster support and increase initiatives to help alleviate suffering. John Paul II teaches that the Christian family is called to give witness of 'generous and disinterested dedication to social matters, through a 'preferential option' for the poor and disadvantaged' (FC 47). He adds that love goes beyond those of the same faith and knows how to discover the face of Christ 'in each individual, especially in the poor, the weak and those who suffer' (FC 64). He admonishes that priests and deacons 'must support the family in its difficulties and sufferings' (FC 73) and that 'a prudent pastoral commitment, modelled on Our Lord, is called for in families which find themselves in difficult situations' (FC 77).

Christ, through his Incarnation, has in a certain way united himself with each human being. He loved with a human heart, and a Christian person 'receives the 'first fruits of the Spirit' (Ro.8.23) by which he is able to fulfil the new law of love' (GS 22). Everyone is, therefore, called to look upon his neighbour as another self, to respect each person, to enable each to live in a dignified way and to come to their aid in a positive way. Jesus laid down the obligation for Christians to treat people as brothers and sisters so that the human race would become the family of God, in which love would be the fullness of the law.

By the Church's very nature and mission, 'she has particularly at heart the lives of the weakest and most sorely tried brothers and sisters' (p518). She recognises Christ in those who are suffering and 'does all in her power to relieve their need and in them she strives to serve Christ' (LG 8).

All Christians are called to the fullness of Christian life and to the perfection of love. The Church teaches that to reach this perfection one must follow in Christ's footsteps in wholehearted devotion to the glory of God and the service of one's neighbour (LG 40); and that love is its characteristic mark. It, therefore, claims charitable works as its mission and right. Wherever people are racked by misfortune or illness, 'Christian charity should comfort them with devoted care and give them the helps that will relieve their needs' (AA 8). Consequently, 'works of mutual aid for the alleviation of all kinds of human needs, are held in special honour in the Church' (AA 8) and today these works of charity have become much more urgent and charitable action should reach all needs (AA 8).

* * *

By early September, I had finishing writing this piece on Church teaching and sent a copy to my tutor. I had found plenty of Church doctrine that I felt was relevant to carers, especially where there is mental illness, and was looking forward to interviewing the clergy and doctor to discover if this teaching was being implemented as well as it might be. Questionnaires were already filtering back to me and I was also looking forward to reading the responses of carers on the issue of Church support.

September proved to be a busy month. Two ladies, Hazel and Joan who, many months previously had contacted me for advice having seen the notice about our support meeting, had been in touch with me again. I had invited them to visit me and while at our house, they had explained that they both suffered a mental illness and wanted more spiritual nourishment. They wondered about starting a group like ours, but for sufferers. Although they attended their own churches, they felt personal prayer and sharing with others who understood would be beneficial to them. I arranged for them to meet Father Joseph and Sister Dierdre, who comes to our group, where we had discussed the issues and prayed together. Father Joseph and I said we would try and come to their first meeting when it was organised.

'So I wondered if you might be coming,' said Hazel, on the telephone. She lived thirty miles away and knew it would be time consuming for Father Joseph and myself to travel. She had sent me a poster with details of the meeting and I had contacted Father Joseph who had written it into his diary.

'Yes, we both hope to be there. I know it's taken many months but you've both done well. It's not easy publicising and visiting places to explain the setting up of something new. We look forward to seeing you both again.' I was delighted for them. It was going to be an ecumenical group entitled: Christian Mental Health Fellowship. We had a good evening with a few gentle songs, a reading from Scripture, a little sharing and some prayer and were served with tea and cake.

It was four days later that my Mam rang. 'I have a pain, Ed It's quite nasty'. It was early Sunday evening and I was just about to go to Mass. We had a short chat. 'I'll ring you back Mam, in an hour,' I said. Mam didn't often complain about pain. When I rang later, she told me she'd been to her doctor's home.

'He just lives over the road; so I thought I'd pop in as the pain was really bad.' I made no comment about her action. She was eighty-two and her reasoning must have made sense to her. Tony had been told and he went along to see Mam. 'I'll ring you tomorrow, Mam,' I said. 'Goodnight and God bless.'

The telephone rang next morning before I was out of bed. 'Ed,' said Mam, 'Can you come? I'm not well?' I looked at the clock. 8.00am. 'Okay, Mam. I'll be along later this morning.'

'What's all that about?' asked Ray as he turned over beside me.' 'It was my Mam. She's not well. I said I would go.' I packed a few bits and pieces and all the questionnaires that had been returned. I thought I might find a few spare moments when I could begin checking and collating the information.

'I don't know how long I might be there,' I said to Ray. We rolled up the foam mattress that was to be my bed, as Mam's home is a one-bedroomed terraced bungalow. Ray drove me the thirty miles to Mam's village, as I wanted to leave my car for Elizabeth. She uses it for work and, although coping, was not fully well.

Mam was violently sick in the early hours of the next morning and it was not a good colour. 'I think it was a real good idea of mine, getting you to come, Ed. Don't you?' she said. 'I do, Mam,' I replied. When her doctor arrived, he was pleased that I was going to stay with her for as long as was needed, and from then on, I was her 'nurse'. I particularly had to make sure she took her medication. We had great banter about her pills because she struggled to swallow them.

'I'm going to write a poem,' she said, 'about a pill.' She held it out on her hand and began. 'Now here is a pill... She was hilarious in spite of being ill. I discovered the extent of her obsessions and had to be very diplomatic about washing clothes and pots. The first time I washed up, Mam stated, 'You haven't put them on there, Ed, have you?' looking at the washed pots on the draining board. 'Mam, I washed it down first. It's all right. You just sit down. I'll be with you in a minute.' She returned to her chair.

We played scrabble and did crosswords and watched television. Mam didn't want me to leave her. Tony called daily and got bits of shopping for us. My brothers and sisters kept turning up at intervals, as well as some of Mam's grandchildren and the telephone kept ringing. There was great concern for our Mam. After I had been there a few days, Paula and Margaret came through from Middlesbrough to see me and we went out for a drink. My Mam didn't really want me to leave her, but Tony had offered to sit with her while I was out. It was a pleasant break for me and really kind of my friends, I thought. Ray turned up with Elizabeth one evening. He brought me some mail, including more completed questionnaires, and I was able to do a little work on them. Elizabeth wasn't so good and was missing me. It was as if she coped as long as she knew I was there for her in case she needed me. We talked on the telephone quite a bit which helped.

The following Monday, early morning, my Mam had another attack of vomiting. Her doctor had been visiting regularly and we were still waiting for the results of tests she had been given at a local hospital. I telephoned the doctor as instructed to do if she vomited again. I was becoming very concerned about Mam. She hadn't eaten for a week and was drinking very little.

'The doctor says he will phone the hospital for the results, Mam, and then come to see you.' Shortly afterwards, he arrived and gave Mam the news. 'I'm afraid you will have to go into hospital for further investigation,' he said and then asked, 'May I use your phone?' 'Of course,' replied Mam. She was always courteous.

'Right, Mam, let's get a bag packed.'

'Why now?' she asked. 'When are we going?'

'As soon as the ambulance comes,' I replied.

'Oh. Oh. But you'll come with me?' she asked.

'Of course, Mam, I'll go in the ambulance with you. I won't leave you.'

'Oh, Ed,' she said, emotionally, and hugged me.

'It's all right,' I said consolingly. 'We'll be okay.' I rang Tony and asked him to let the family know.

It was a long journey for Mam, thirty miles in the ambulance, but she just cracked jokes with the drivers and complimented them on their work. No sooner had we arrived at the hospital than Miriam turned up. 'I'm so glad to see you,' I said.

'I got the message from Tony and came straight here. It's only a few minutes on the bus for me,' replied Miriam. Grace also arrived shortly after Miriam. Lucky Mam with three daughters round her bed. Mam was put in a side ward and soon there were nurses and doctors around asking many questions.

'Mam, Grace and I are going now,' I said, when she was settled in. We left her after hugs and kisses and Grace took me back to Mam's bungalow. I rolled up my mattress, collected together my few belongings and my paperwork and waited for Tony's arrival. He had offered to take me back to Middlesbrough where I knew there were more traumas awaiting.

14
REVIEW OF LITERATURE: CARING, ESPECIALLY THOSE WITH MENTAL ILLNESS

It was a good feeling to be back in my own bed on the Monday night after a week away, but I wasn't sleeping so well because of other family tragedies. Sara, aged twenty-two, the daughter of my niece Susan, had been taken into a hospice to have her medication for pain regulated. Sara had had four operations over the last two years and was seriously ill with cancer. Susan's other daughter, Anne, aged twenty-one, had been in hospital with serious head injuries since being a passenger in a car crash in June 1996, and was still in hospital, unable to talk, walk, or feed herself. There had been some improvement in her condition as she was now smiling. These two girls used to stay with us when children and Jonathan and Elizabeth had spent some holidays with them. As there were plenty of family to visit my Mam, I felt that I could give some support to my niece.

Susan was at the hospice when I arrived. We went out on to the balcony and had a cigarette and chat. As well as being my goddaughter, Susan was my Mam's oldest grandchild and I was able to update her on Mam's condition. She likewise shared her news on her two daughters. After Anne's accident two years ago, I had been a regular visitor to the hospital in which she was being cared for and Ray and I had often visited her. The hospice was situated next to the hospital where Anne was looked after, which was convenient for Susan as she was able to bring Anne in a wheel chair to join visitors around Sara's bedside.

'I must go now,' I said to Susan. Jacqueline's first baby is due any day and I want to make sure all is well with her.'

I telephoned Jacqueline as soon as I arrived home and she reassured me that she was fine. I spent a little time working on my dissertation. I wanted to complete some of the literature review and post it to my tutor for his comments. It had been quite a task putting all the research literature material together in a coherent whole as there was material referring to carers in general and some specifically to carers of people with mental illness.

* * *

Carers

There are many categories of carers, but, in this review of literature on carers, the emphasis is on the understanding that the word 'carer' means anyone unpaid who looks after a relative or friend unable to manage without help as cited by the author Ledger. This review also has particular emphasis on the role of caring where there is mental illness. Both Ledger (1992) and Burton-Jones (1992: 16) state that carers are ordinary people who come from all educational backgrounds and social groups. Burton-Jones feels that society needs to acknowledge the tremendous upheaval carers face 'in taking on accountability for a sick loved one'. McCann (1995: 12) believes that 'the foundation of care is respect' and that this includes both self-respect and respect for the unique dignity of the individually cared for person.

Carer literature

Kohner (1992) says that carers have much in common. Perring *et al* (1994), Burton-Jones (1992), Twigg and Atkin (1994), and Atkinson and Coia (1995) all make the point that persons diagnosed as suffering from mental illness demand a different kind of caring to those with physical disability, a very important observation. Perring *et al* explain that the need for care of a dependant with learning difficulties is most likely to have existed since birth, whereas mental illness usually begins in adolescence or adulthood. In re-examining literature on families caring for people diagnosed as mentally ill, they found that carer literature had tended to concentrate on carers of people needing physical support, while carers of people suffering mental illness had been neglected and Wainright (1997) agrees with this. They add that, even in the separate development of literature in psychiatric and psychological fields, these carers had tended to be marginalised and only rarely looked at in their own right. Hogman and

Pearson (1995: 3) state that policy makers, health and local authorities, have known these needs for years but 'they just have not been given a high enough priority' and Twigg and Atkin (1994) and Stobbart (1996) have similar concerns.

Care in the Community

Care in the community, a result of a policy leading to the eventual closing of long-stay hospitals and of developing community-based services, implies a major increase in responsibility for families where a member suffers a mental illness; and they face considerable difficulties says Perring *et al.* Wainright (1997: 70) states that 'the burden of care in the community rests more heavily on their shoulders than ever before' and is asking for consideration of the effects that this has on the families' physical, emotional and financial resources. These carers, in terms of priority for local authority funding, have been 'pushed to the back of the queue' declare Twigg and Atkin (1994:114) and their needs are neglected, as they are seen as a natural resource, thus saving the government billions of pounds, a fact made by Burton-Jones (1992) and Hogman and Pearson (1995). Wainright believes that, in the fight for resources, these carers are an inevitable early casualty. Hogman and Pearson say that, rather than these carers being valued, they are taken for granted and have been discriminated against when caring at home, as statutory services are more available if the ill person moves out. They believe that these carers should be respected and their needs recognised. 'It is time to secure more support for the families of the mentally ill' says Wallace (1996: 3).

Loss of personality

Burton-Jones points out that an area that causes much distress to carers, is that they can find it hurtful and difficult to tolerate the attitude of the sufferer through the personality changes the illness brings about, especially in mental illness. Perring *et al* state that it can seem as if the carer is 'living with a completely different person' (1990: 11). Jee and Reason (1988) feel that this personality change brings out a great sense of sadness in the carer and is akin to a bereavement in the loss of a person they once knew, a point made by Kohner (1992), Ledger (1992), Burton-Jones (1992) and Twigg and Atkin (1994). Wainright (1997) feels that this is a particularly painful experience because of the damage to the relationship. It is as if the attachment bond is not broken, but violated and the carer emotionally abused as the sufferer speaks and behaves in a way unimaginable in the past.

Stress on family life

McCann (1995) found that stress on a carer is heightened because responsibility tends to fall consistently on one individual in the family, particularly where there is mental illness. Perring *et al* (1994), Twigg and Atkin (1994) and Atkinson and Coia (1995: 92) all make this point. Atkinson and Coia state that 'there is very little evidence to support the notion of a caring community' and suggest that care in the community is, in reality, the family. There are considerable levels of disruption to family life where there is mental illness (Perring *et al*, 1994; Moate and Enoch, 1990). Twigg and Atkin find that marriage ties are weakened, and Perring *et al* that many families do not remain intact and there is a high level of marital breakdown.

Burton-Jones believes that the greatest demands on the carer are from within the household, as family members are affected and many carers feel particularly that they are letting down their other children. Living with this tension in relationships, she says, 'can be intolerable' (Burton-Jones, 1992: 82). My research shows that this is an area where carers' support groups can be of help in that feelings can be expressed and tension released outside the family situation. Perring *et al* state that emphasis on the family's well-being in its own right is a comparatively recent interest. A person with mental illness can become increasingly demanding of their family which 'can act as a severe restraint on the carer's own life', but that 'the impact for the primary carer has not generally been addressed' (Perring *et al*, 1994: 9,13).

Isolation

Perring *et al* declare that this restraint on a carer's own life is evident in that social life for the carer is shown to be severely restricted and, as Moate and Enoch (1990: 111) affirm, leads to isolation between the family 'and the rest of the world around', or as Hogman and Pearson (1995) and Stobbart (1996) state, to isolation from family and friends. Burton-Jones (1992: 87) states that the carer feels rejected and lonely when friends distance themselves and adds that 'when two-thirds of carers recently interviewed said that no-one ever listened to them, it seems to sum up what carers feel about this isolation'. She believes that thoughtless remarks from outside the family demonstrate the lack of understanding of the carer's situation; and that no-one sees it as being necessary to ask how the carer is feeling.

She gives two reasons for this lack of understanding; that empathy for the carer can be very painful and that for much of their lives, carers are invisible. Ledger (1992: 129) declares that this 'isolation from others is a common, very painful, experience for carers', and Kohner agrees. McCann says that it 'can be one of the carer's deepest sufferings' (McCann, 1995: 36). McCann also states that the carers in the home 'have held the Cinderella position within the whole field of caring' and that family carers go largely unnoticed even though their contribution to caring is enormous; and that they provide the bulk of the care in this country.

Stigma

An outcome of this lack of understanding, Burningham (1989) cites, is that carers of people suffering mental illness are likely to see their situation as something of which to be ashamed and to be hidden from the outside world. 'Ignorance and fear are two powerful forces that have prevented the advancement of care' declare Moate and Enoch (1990: 85) for both sufferers and carers. Perring *et al* (1990), Carson (1992) and Stobbart (1996) all agree that some carers avoid contact with friends and neighbours because of shame and fear of stigma. Twigg and Atkin (1994) state that the social isolation imposed, where there are mental health problems in family life, reinforces guilt and stigma and is particularly distressing for relatives, also reported by Perring et al and, in general, carers 'feel that they have to cope with a world that does not want to understand their situation' (Perring *et al*, 1994: 106).

Hogman and Pearson find that ignorance and misunderstanding can bring additional pain and difficulties for families. Atkinson and Coia state that 'mental illness has always been stigmatised, and both people with the condition and their relatives have been isolated' (Atkinson and Coia, 1995: 128). They add that this has come about, and still does, from a largely ill-informed public. Wallace (1996: 5) feels that the media publicity on violent incidents, although inevitably and properly reported, generates stigma and the only way to reduce this is to 'explain why they are happening and to campaign for better help for the sufferer and understanding for families and victims' .

'Stigma,' Wainright (1997: 50) declares, 'remains a reality'. These findings powerfully reinforce my own belief that stigma and shame are still strongly felt by sufferers of mental illness and their families.

Emotional stress

Hogman and Pearson (1995) and Stobbart (1996) find that the illness of the sufferer has totally changed some carers' lives because, without support, their effectiveness as carers deteriorates, and when they lose contact with family and friends, their health is affected. Wainright (1997: 175) speaks of 'an overwhelming emotional pain', which comes partly from watching their loved one suffer and Kupiers *et al* (1989: 775) state that 'emotional demands on relatives who provide support for those in continuous and intensive contact with psychiatric services may continue for years'. Almost three quarters of relatives suffer psychiatric symptoms or physical ill-health state Perring *et al* (1994) and Burton-Jones (1992) and they find their very high level of psychiatric distress is three times greater than the community norm. Moate and Enoch (1990) speak of carers having feelings of helplessness and hopelessness and Jee and Reason (1988) report of great inner tension and guilt. In spite of all this, Atkinson and Coia (1995) say there is very little research on the psychology of care. Swinton and Kettles (1997: 118) suggest that, 'the act of caring may well become neglected and subsumed by the emphasis on empirical research data to validate and legitimate our own professional status'.

Financial hardship; respite care

A further area of concern among carers is that many eventually, through the continual demands of caring, have to resign from work and suffer a fall in family income and consequent financial deprivation (Moate and Enoch, 1990; Burton-Jones, 1992). Perring *et al* (1994) and Hogman and Pearson (1995) find that the majority of studies investigating financial situations of carers have found that they have difficulties in this area, which are directly related to having a member of the family suffering mental illness. A support that would clearly benefit carers financially, as well as health-wise, is that of respite care, which Hogman and Pearson found wanted by nearly three-quarters of carers. They state that it is essential that carers be given a break from caring as does Kohner (1992). However, respite is 'almost totally absent as a concept within the mental health sector' (Twigg and Atkinson, 1994: 116).

Support groups

According to McCann (1995), carers' support groups are particularly helpful because of the support carers give to each other and Kupiers *et al* (1989) say, are cost-effective support for carers. These are 'one of the most positive developments in the mental health field in recent years' says Burningham (1989: 144). Atkinson and Coia (1995: 115; 128) state that 'all self-help groups engage in education' for the individuals taking part and also are aimed at the general public to heighten awareness of carers' problems and to reduce the stigma. They add that the groups first arose 'out of a deep need of relatives to share their burden with an unknowing and unconcerned world' and also to receive support and understanding. They note that 'it maybe a testimony to the despair felt by relatives that they would brave this stigma to meet others in the same position'.

Burningham (1989), Kupiers (1989) and Carson (1992) find that self-help and support groups help overcome the feeling of stigma and shame. A very important element in helping people to cope is in the discovery, and the understanding that comes from this, of those who have the same problems, a point made by Burningham (1989), McCarthy *et al* (1989), Kohner (1992), Carson (1992) and Atkinson and Coia (1995). McCann (1995) and Kupiers *et al* (1989) believe that support groups help prevent feelings of isolation, give a sense of perspective, improve coping abilities, and provide a social outlet. McCarthy *et al* find they are non-judgmental environments of acceptance and support where carers can share pent-up difficult feelings especially of guilt, anger and grief (McCarthy *et al*, 1989; Kupiers *et al*, 1989).

'A self-help support group is a life-line to many', states Ledger (1992: 143), a point affirmed by Stobbart. However, Wainright found that some carers did not wish to meet others similarly situated, as they felt barely able to cope with their own family, whereas Hogman and Pearson find carers' contact with their peers, who can share experiences and give support, is a vital part of community care. While a counselling and support group is not able to meet the needs of all relatives, McCarthy *et al*, Kupiers *et al*, and Carson and Stobbart all believe that this sort of group ought to become a routine part of service offered by the community care facilities. Atkinson and Coia (1995: 131) inform us that 'the magnitude and importance of the support, which comes from these groups, is difficult to comprehend for people who are not themselves involved'. Hogman and Pearson state that service providers and purchasers ought to build up their relationships with carer groups. There is much confirmation here of my own belief that support groups give a good measure of help to carers.

Spiritual Support

Carers have many different needs and Swinton and Kettles feel that an approach to an individual needs to respect the person holistically, as one with physical, emotional and spiritual needs. I was very pleased to find this point made as it was the kind of approach that I had needed. They add that when people's spirituality is taken into full account, they are seen as people rather than problems and this approach embodies respect for persons because 'a person's spirituality is the overarching framework within which a person interprets and makes sense of their reality' (Swinton and Kettles, 1997: 119). McCann, too, sees basic human needs as divided into physical, intellectual, emotional and spiritual. Atkinson and Coia (1995) refer to Pratt *et al* who report that Levine *et al* found carers 'with an internal locus of control tended to cope better', and that Pratt *et al* name spiritual support as one of two aids associated with significantly less carer burden.

However, Moate and Enoch (1990: 111) state that lack of understanding from church members accentuates the difficulties of relatives; that there be must particular concern about lack of support by Christian Churches where there is mental illness; and that church members 'often became hostile and discontinued the past friendship' when a friend's son or daughter developed a severe mental illness. Nolan and Crawford (1997: 293) state that it is the special carers who give attention twenty-four hours daily within the community care model of today, and that they are often the family members of the person suffering mental illness. They add that 'in order to make these relationships effective for the client and sustainable by the carer, nurses need to be active in supporting the families of mentally ill people... Nurses have also to extend their understanding of the aetiology of mental illness and educate others about mental health from the perspective of the spiritual needs of the community'. Benefits of spirituality, Swinton and Kettles (1997: 119) state, include offering hope, meaning and a purposeful future and 'binding to community [all of] which are often omitted from caring strategies'.

Spiritual pain is a profound reality that, 'may be the pain that requires most attention and help [and] concerns the depth of what it means to be human,' (McCann, 1995: 113). I thought this an excellent point and most affirming. Burton-Jones (1992: 61–62) says that the many tears shed 'reveal how close to the surface streams a well of relentless grief, anger and despair' and feels that these feelings are 'part of a person's spiritual response to a human tragedy'. She adds that, 'while the emotional level can be alleviated, some carers need the spiritual dimension exploring'. McCann (1995: 56) believes that 'everyone has profound spiritual needs' and, although lying below the surface of the carer's consciousness, will inevitably surface and may do so with great force.

'The pain of profound experience can be increased if there isn't anyone around to help the sufferer' (McCann 1995: 114). Nolan and Crawford state that 'the language of spirituality provides a way of talking about meaning and purpose' (Nolan and Crawford, 1997: 291–3) and refer to Frankl, who stated that to be human is to be constantly searching for meaning. They continue that people are at a key stage in this search when in a crisis and that 'this call for a rhetoric of spirituality is to ensure that the spiritual is valued alongside the scientific'.

All this research reinforcing the need of spiritual support was very encouraging. I do believe that the Church has a role to fulfil in its mission of love in action where there is mental illness, and there are many points made here as a reminder to the Church. It has the means to offer healing to people suffering and in need.

Facts of caring

There are those carers who believe that caring can bring its own rewards (Jee and Reason, 1988; Ledger, 1992; Burton-Jones, 1992). Perring *et al* find that some want to care for their dependants, but others do not. Hogman and Pearson highlight this as an important factor and go on to point out that carers have individual needs, that they are experts in severe mental illness, and that their requests for services are at a minimum in comparison with their needs. They state that 'it is a sad reflection on our society that caring families are more likely to see the police than a whole section of the service, which should be available for the care of people with a severe mental illness and their families' (Hogman and Pearson, 1995: 31).

In conclusion, in the provision of services, Twigg and Atkin feel that carers tend to be neglected. Hogman and Pearson believe that they want respect for their work and for their experience. McCann lists requirements needed by the family carer: that of recognition and status; of education and support; of community-based health, social and educational facilities; and respite care facilities. Hogman and Pearson and Stobbart state that carers' knowledge of severe mental illness is an important resource and they feel their own needs for services should be respected. Hogman and Pearson (1995: 46) conclude that the praiseworthy attempts to treat sufferers more humanely in the community have been undermined by lack of resources and an infrastructure. Meanwhile, they conclude that carers have now become the isolated ones, 'the Silent Partners in community care'. I conclude this review with Ledger's comment that 'the only really long-lasting hope that can be offered to carers is the hope there is in Jesus Christ' (Ledger, 1992: 137).

* * *

I felt quite overwhelmed by reading this literature. Over and over again, I was identifying with the views expressed and I was delighted to be reassured that nourishment of a carer's spirituality is seen to be important, in fact almost essential for the well-being of the person. It would appear that the greater the suffering a carer experiences, the more important the need for support and, where there is mental illness, suffering of the carer is acknowledged as being intensified. I managed to put this chapter of my dissertation in the post before I had to put my studying on hold because of family events, which began accumulating. Shortly I would be grieving the loss of two close relatives.

15
REVIEW OF LITERATURE: CARERS' PERSONAL EXPERIENCES

As September 1997 was drawing to a close, events in my life were escalating. I made another visit to the hospice to find little change in Sara's condition and the messages from my brothers and sisters about Mam had not been good. There was no improvement in her condition and the consultant had decided to operate. On Saturday Mam would go down to theatre. I worried about her because she was only seven and a half stone and eighty-two years old. Mam needed the operation to put right a blockage in her bowel that was life-threatening.

'Mam, it's Jacqueline. Can you come. My waters have broken.' It was 7.30pm on the Friday evening. I drove to her house, a few streets away. She was putting her bags into the car. Anthony, her partner's ten-year-old needed looking after. 'I'll just stay by the phone,' I said, smiling. 'Good luck.' I gave Jacqueline a big hug. It is a waiting game when a baby is imminent. Anthony finally went to bed at ten o'clock and it was just after midnight when the telephone rang. A boy. I was delighted for them and went to bed. It was in the early hours that I heard Dave, Jacqueline's partner, come home. At about six o'clock, there was a knock on my bedroom door.

'Do you want a cup of tea, Edna?' It was Dave. He stood and talked at length about the birth of his baby boy who had a mass of black hair.

'I'll go now, Dave,' I said. 'I'll go in to see Jacqueline later. I was picking up her washing from the hospital. A gran's job.

Later that morning I phoned the hospital where my Mam was. She was back from theatre.

'But will there be any point in coming tonight?' I asked. The nurse reassured me that I could go.

'Would you mind?' I asked Ray, but I knew he wouldn't. So we went the journey of about sixty miles because I hadn't seen Mam since Monday and I did want to see her so much. I hardly recognised her in the ward. A little, old, frail, grey-haired lady with a mask on her ashen face.

'Oh, Mam,' I whispered as I tried to hold her. Her arms came up and she smiled with her eyes.

'Oh, Mam,' is all I could say. I sat beside her bed and held her hand while a few tears rolled down my cheeks.

'Never mind, Mam,' I said. 'It's over now and we'll soon be back home playing scrabble again. You might even beat me,' I joked. She drifted over into sleep and I crept away. As I reached the door of the ward, I glanced back at her. My poor Mam. Then it was back home again.

Elizabeth and I went to the hospice on Sunday. Sara lay in bed looking pale and thin. She was drifting in and out of sleep. She opened her eyes.

'Hello, Elizabeth,' she said quietly. 'How are you doing?'

'I'm all right. I'm doing fine,' Elizabeth replied. I had had many conversations with Sara when visiting her after her operations, or meeting up when visiting Anne and she had taken a great interest in Elizabeth's illness. Afterwards Elizabeth said to me, 'How could she, Mam? How could she ask about me when she is so ill herself?' It was one of the last things Sara said.

'You ought to let Jonathan know how ill Sara is,' Elizabeth said to me when we got back home on Sunday evening.

'I have told him, but I will ring him tonight,' I replied. 'She is really very ill. I don't know how much longer we'll have her.' I could see Elizabeth was struggling over Sara. Jonathan would be a support for her too. I returned on Monday to the hospice. Sara fell asleep for the last time and slipped into a coma.

Many visitors came and went. At about 11.30pm, Ray walked in with Jonathan. He had come all the way from Liverpool to visit Sara. I hugged him.

'You can speak to her. The hearing is the last thing to go,' I said. He went to her bedside and I could hear whispers. My heart bled for him. We left after midnight. Elizabeth was waiting up for us. A few minutes later, she said to me, 'I think someone might need you, Mam,' as she pointed to the kitchen. I glanced over and saw Jonathan silently sobbing, his shoulders heaving. I went and held him.

'All the way home from Liverpool on the bus Mam, I was planning my conversation with Sara and now it's too late', he said, fighting his tears. As has happened many times before when writing this book, I can hardly see the keyboard for the tears, which stream down my face. I ached for my son. Watching someone dying isn't an easy experience for anyone, let alone a young person.

Before returning to the hospice later on Tuesday, I went to bring Jacqueline and our latest grandchild home from hospital. I settled her in her house with Dave there to look after her. My sister Grace, Susan's mother, had been staying at the hospice with Susan, while Grace's husband looked after Sara's two little ones. Sara was a single parent Mum and soon her two children would be without a mother. Susan had brought Anne over from the hospital.

'You know,' Susan said to us, 'I have two daughters and now neither of them can talk to me.' On Wednesday evening after the departure of many visitors, Grace, Susan and myself were round Sara's bed. Her breathing changed and we knew. We prayed together quietly watching, waiting, listening.

'She's going,' I whispered. Her little gasps for breath were becoming weaker and weaker. It's as if time stands still. A last little puff of air and then she was gone. To experience death is a sacred moment for me when I am privileged to be present at the meeting of this world and the next. It is awesome. It was 11.20pm.

Well after midnight, Susan decided to go and spend the night with her parents and grandchildren. She wanted to give Sara's children the news in person. So I found myself praying my way home at 2.30am having driven Susan and Grace the thirty miles to Grace's home over the moors. Luckily there was little traffic about at such an hour because I was really on overdrive. In the car, we had discussed the fact that someone was going to have to tell Mam that her great granddaughter had died. Susan decided that she would like to tell her Gran, herself.

'Oh, Ed, have you come to take me home?' These were Mam's opening words when I arrived on the Saturday evening.

'I can't, Mam. You're not well enough,' I replied. Ray decided he would go and get a cup of tea and Jonathan and

Elizabeth went with him, 'But you can't go,' said Mam. 'You stay with me.'

'I don't mind that at all, Mam,' I said smiling at her. 'I love you, Mam.' We stayed till the end of visiting time. I was reluctant to leave Mam. Thinking about her on the way home, I felt most concerned. I hadn't seen her for a week and I sensed that something was not right.

On arriving home, even though it was late, I rang two of my sisters to see how they saw the situation only to find that they too were worried. 'I'll ring the consultant on Monday,' I told them, 'and make an appointment to see him.' I went to bed uneasy. The telephone call never took place as we were all called to the hospital on Sunday evening.

Mam had taken a turn for the worse. She was back in a side ward. Her seven children all arrived together with five of their spouses. Tony called the priest and we all prayed. After midnight, we were asked to leave apart from two or three at the most and after discussion, three of us stayed all night seated on chairs round Mam's bed. My brother and sister left early next morning. Ray had slept in the car all night and came in to see me and Mam. Mam gesticulated that she wanted to write something. At this point she wasn't speaking much. Ray went out and bought an exercise book for her and produced a pen. Mam wrote messages in this book in scrawly, wavering writing that I struggled to decipher. She asked had Ray had his breakfast. She asked if Father Joseph was coming to see her. I had telephoned him and he hoped to come. She loved him and considered him her best friend.

Ray left for home and Mam was moved to the intensive care ward and there was talk of further surgery. She beckoned for her writing book and wrote, 'no crucifix in here?' I rang one of the family and later a sister-in-law brought one in, which Mam held constantly. Mam now had one or more of her children with her at all times. I hadn't left the hospital and on the Monday evening I was asked to call all close relatives using the telephone from the relatives room, which I thought very kind of the nurse. In ones and twos they came and we waited. At ten o'clock at night, the consultant came in and explained that a further operation was not possible and we knew it was the beginning of the end.

Next morning Mam came out of a deep sleep and talked of the joy of where she was going. It was a privilege to listen.

Miriam and I were overjoyed. Then Tony came and Mam awoke again and told him. Later Father Joseph came to see her and her eyes lit up. It was so good to see him. It was wonderful for Mam. Mam was moved from intensive care to a side room on another ward, as it was a question of finding a bed for her, and the family continued with round the clock visiting. I stayed until Friday. Those few days were happy ones. Mam's illness had disappeared. She laughed and joked and was wonderful company. She was so alive, so animated. It was as if her real personality was back. She was such a joy. She knew she was dying, but she was so happy. One night about midnight, there were five of us children round her bed trying to recall 'There's a one-eyed yellow idol', one of Mam's party pieces. There we were putting in the actions too. A nurse popped her head round the door. 'Having a party in here?' she asked jokingly.

On the doctors' round on Thursday morning, a little entourage of four came into Mam's room. I was on my own with Mam as Amy had left at 6.30am and Miriam was due to arrive at any time.

'Would you like to go home, Muriel?' the doctor asked her. Mam looked at me. 'Do you mean for me to take her home and look after her?' I asked. The doctor answered, 'Yes.'

'Mam,' I asked, 'would you like to come home to my house and I'll look after you?' Her face lit up. 'Oh, yes,' she replied.

'Guess what?' I said to Miriam when she arrived a few minutes later, 'I can take Mam home.' I passed the news on to my brothers and sisters. Lots of arrangements had to be made including ringing my own doctor to ask if he would oversee Mam's care. The outcome was that I would go home on Friday and return on Sunday to travel the sixty miles journey on Monday with Mam by ambulance. 'Bye, Mam. See you Sunday, I said, giving her a big hug. I wanted her to spend her last days surrounded by her family at home.

But before Sunday, we had Saturday to get through. It was Sara's funeral Mass. In the little village, the church was packed. Susan had Sara's two children with her and a friend of Susan's had brought Anne the thirty miles so that she could attend her sister's funeral. Cousins had made the journey from various parts of the country and then went back knowing that in a short time they would be recalled for Mam's funeral. Jonathan had stayed for the funeral, but returned to Liverpool after seeing Mam in our home on the Monday. It had seemed a long and bumpy ride for Mam. I could see, sitting beside her in the ambulance, that she was finding it stressful, but she made no complaint. I had prepared our home for her over the weekend with the help of my family. There were beautiful flowers awaiting her when we arrived, a personal touch from Stephanie.

Two weeks later in the same church, we celebrated again the life of a loved one. All our eight children and four grandchildren were present. Jacqueline had told me to tell Mam to hang on and see her baby and she had. We had Mam in our house for eight days again with round the clock watching by her children and their spouses. Father Joseph had visited her a number of times and concelebrated at her funeral Mass. Father Desmond, who had visited Elizabeth when she had had her first relapse, also came to see Mam at my house. Mam loved this. Our doctor visited a number of times. I felt we were very fortunate to have such care and attention and I was immensely grateful to my doctor and the priests. The day nurses and the twilight nurses were also exceedingly kind and attentive. On their last visit on the Monday evening, one of them said, 'She's very poorly. We'll disturb her as little as possible.'

I knew the end was coming. Grace and I stayed with her all night. Shortly after midnight she opened her eyes for the last time and gave a radiant smile. She was so happy. She quietly left us next morning at 9.40am. I cried. I loved her. I wished more people could be allowed to die surrounded by such love and care as my Mam had received over those last days.

I was very busy the week after Mam's funeral, giving me little time to grieve. I went to the carers' meeting at St Thomas More's on the Thursday evening. It was good to share about my Mam and I found it helpful. On Saturday, I had to travel to York, an hour's drive, to speak at the Annual General Meeting of the Association of Pastoral Care in Mental Health. I was ill-prepared because of all the happenings at home over the last weeks, but the offer by a friend to take me made the day more bearable.

It was in the weeks to come when I found myself thinking about my Mam that I began to feel angry. I went to see my doctor first and then talked with Father Joseph. 'Father Joseph,' I explained, 'my Mam could have had such a better quality of life if she hadn't kept her illness so hidden. She suffered for years and years and if society had had a different attitude towards people with these illnesses, Mam wouldn't have felt so different. She could have received help and sympathy as with other illnesses, but it had to be kept so hidden. She didn't want people thinking she was odd or strange.'

My resolve to finish my dissertation was even stronger. It had been put on hold for weeks, but now I wanted to work at it again and I gathered together the literature I had located on carers' personal experiences, some with special reference to mental illness. I wrote a review on it.

* * *

Carers

One carer's definition of what it is to be a carer is of 'someone who understands, and loves and cares, irrespective of illness' (Dean, 1995: 16).

Loss of personality

A carer's description of this loss is that 'it is as though your child dies... but you don't have to contend with death, you have to contend with transformation' (Edginton, 1993: 13). Another carer says that she felt a sense of loss of a part of her son when schizophrenia was diagnosed and that the biggest heartache was that their son 'was becoming a stranger to us' (Moate and Enoch, 1990: 42).

I remember walking into our kitchen one day and saying to Elizabeth, 'It's like we've got you back, the lovely Elizabeth that we knew.' Her personality was shining through again.

Stress on family life

A carer explains that she and her husband rarely went out and 'had drifted into a meaningless existence' (Jubilee Centre, 1990: 28). Another carer states that she and her husband were at loggerheads and no longer got together with other people (Edginton, 1993). The family of a sufferer became isolated individuals, desperate and confused (Edginton, 1993). One carer describes her family relationships as being strained at times and that their lives have changed (Arkless, 1995). Another found problems with her three older children and 'feels teenagers and young adults have a problem understanding mental illness' (McCann, 1995: 108). The same carer's marriage almost broke; the stress was enormous (McCann, 1995).

Isolation

A carer speaks of feeling despair and also of isolation when friends no longer visited. She says that carers need friendship, contacts and support to deal with the stress and trauma (Jubilee Centre, 1990). Another carer gave up her job to care for her mother and eventually outside activities ceased. She says that 'over the months I had become completely isolated. I was no longer a person, just a caring machine' (Jubliee Centre, 1990: 27). A carer suffered 'a time of great isolation' (Caplin, 1993: 11) during the first years of her son's illness. She felt trapped in another world with him 'but because you love them you cannot let go of the hope that they will change back into the person they were'. Another carer with a son who has been sectioned four times, declares that most friends prefer to stay away and that 'cards and gifts are also usually non-existent' (Arkless, 1995: 15).

My experience as a carer is that meeting together in empathy with other carers helped address these very deep feelings of isolation that I had experienced.

Stigma

One carer's main problem was coming to terms with the knowledge that a member of their family had a severe mental illness (McCann, 1995). A carer declares that before diagnosis, her worst fear was that it might be mental illness; that she was filled with horror of the word 'schizophrenia', 'this terrible scourge called mental illness' (Moate and Enoch, 1990: 47, 55) and that anyone who has experienced mental illness at close proximity 'will realise the full horror of it'.

Emotional stress

A carer sums up her life as 'hard; physically demanding and emotionally draining... It is a kind of prison' (Jubilee Centre, 1990: 4), while another expresses it as 'essentially a matter of emotional and mental stress' (Jubilee Centre, 1990: 8). Another carer states how difficult it was 'to put into words our feelings of utter helplessness and despair' (Moate and Enoch, 1990: 54). Yet another speaks of the 'dark' days when she first began caring; of the sleepless nights, terrified that (her son) would take his own life. She talks of the agony of watching his intense struggle to survive and of his changed personality; this a period of 'sheer desperation' (Schram, 1995: 13). And another carer says that many people not involved in mental illness 'cannot comprehend the heartache and worry' (Dean, 1995: 15) that caring can cause. One carer talks about 'crying, every single day' (Edginton, 1993: 12) and eventually tried to commit suicide. Another carer who is conscious of needing respite care himself, at one point contemplated suicide (Card, 1995). Yet another who had reached the end of her resources 'both physically and emotionally' (Ledger, 1992: 48) was rescued through a friend recommending a break, demonstrating how important is respite care.

Support groups

A carer, while feeling it a privilege to care for her mother, needed outside help to survive and joined a carers group which gave her outside interest (Jubilee Centre, 1990). A carer feels that relatives' needs must be addressed in the same way as those people in mental stress and she and others set up a relatives support group and says that 'we have a long list of grievances' (Edginton, 1993: 13). It was in the support groups that, for the first time, I met with others whom I felt understood what I had experienced and empathised with me.

Spiritual Support.

Ledger tells of a carer who believes that carers in general have been neglected, that although Christians are excellent in the short-term response, 'even in a lively, thriving church, both carer and sick person can begin to feel lonely and isolated' (Ledger, 1992: 43), which causes tension. He says that he could not cope and although he received practical help from his church, he was affected by people asking after his wife, but never himself. He longed for someone to show concern and love for him. Eventually fellow leaders helped him through his tears to see that God does care. When much needed support, including practical help, was received from the wider Christian family, it became one of the main factors that enabled another carer, who was almost at breaking point, and her family, to survive. The carer explained that it was particularly the practical support that was appreciated, especially of one person for 'her sensitivity to us for showing her Christian faith in this practical way' (Ledger, 1992: 22).

A carer speaks of her tears and of not being able to pray in such a dark time (Moate and Enoch, 1990). Another, who suffered grief, anger and resentment in the loss of her 'normal' baby after its being diagnosed as 'mentally handicapped', felt 'very unsupported both emotionally and practically' (Ledger, 1992: 36) even though friends were praying for her. She had feelings of despair and longed for someone to help bear her burdens. She felt rejected and hurt and needed to be listened to. Later she discovered that church members had not fully understood the intensity of her grief and had felt inadequate and unsure about her handicapped child. Her general practitioner, a Christian, was very supportive, as were two friends in a practical way. She states that emotional, spiritual and practical support are so important and that the Church can help in encouragement, prayer and practical help (Ledger, 1992).

It was in the depths of my emptiness and pain that I needed spiritual nourishment beyond any emotional or psychological support being received, and our Church Scripture-based support group particularly helped in addressing this need. Finally, carers, who experience deep spiritual needs, need them addressing. This need I described as a longing 'for a compassionate Christ to walk with us as I journeyed with my daughter in her pain' (Hunneysett, 1994).

* * *

During the writing of this review, I had identified many times with the statements of individual carers. My belief, when Elizabeth was very ill, that there must be others suffering like me had been born out by the insights that these carers had revealed. I was pleased to have another part of my dissertation completed. My next step was to examine and collate the responses from the questionnaires returned by the carers and analyse the information.

Meanwhile Elizabeth had been struggling with the death of Sara and then of her Gran. She had been close to my Mam. They had been bonded in a special way because of their illnesses, even though the diagnoses were different and they had often talked to each other on the telephone. Mam used to send Elizabeth crossword books to pass the time when she was ill. I wondered if Elizabeth's health would be adversely affected because of the deaths within days of two people whom she knew well. She was making good progress at work and had been taken on full-time the week before Mam had died. There was also promotion on the horizon for her. She was skilled at her job. Little did I know that there was another shock waiting for us round the corner.

16
ANALYSIS OF CARERS' QUESTIONNAIRES

One Sunday morning, now early December 1997, I answered the telephone and a voice said, 'Hello, Mam, it's Jacqueline. Are you in for the next half hour?'

'Yes,' I answered.

'I'll be round shortly,' she said.

'Okay,' I replied.' I wonder what that is all about,' I thought. Within ten minutes, Jacqueline arrived with her baby, Barnaby. He was asleep and she placed his carrycot in the back room where we study and relax without the TV. She went into the kitchen and spoke quietly with Elizabeth before coming through to the lounge.

'Mam, can you come upstairs for a few minutes, please?' I sensed an uneasiness in her approach and had a foreboding feeling inside of me. I went upstairs and Jacqueline called, 'We're in here, Mam.' Elizabeth was sitting on my bed with Jacqueline standing. Jacqueline looked at Elizabeth and looked at me. 'Elizabeth has something to tell you Mam,' she said. I looked at Elizabeth.

'I'm having a baby', she said quietly, watching to see my reaction.

I sat down on the bed beside Elizabeth, put my arm round her and said, 'It'll be all right. We'll look after you.' Elizabeth looked tense. 'We'll all give you lots of support,' Jacqueline added and turning to me, said, 'Elizabeth has been wanting to tell you, Mam, but she didn't want to give you any more worry until you had finished your current piece of dissertation writing because you were getting so stressed out with it, especially after Gran and Sara dying. She knew you had a deadline to keep.'

'That was really thoughtful of you, Elizabeth,' I replied. We were all talking quite normally and quietly. No-one would ever have guessed that I had just been hit by a thunderbolt. My thoughts were swirling round and round in my head.

'Have you been to the doctor's, Elizabeth, and had the baby confirmed?' I asked.

'I saw him on Tuesday and he asked if I'd told you, but I explained I was waiting until you'd finished your piece of writing. He said that that was very considerate of me. But I was upset. He suggested I talk to Jacqueline because she'd just had a baby.'

'And when's the baby due then?' I asked.

'At the beginning of August,' Elizabeth replied. She stood up and I put my arms round her. She must be feeling so scared, I thought. 'I've been wanting to tell you, Mam.'

'Well, it's all right now,' I answered. We went downstairs because Elizabeth wanted to tell her Dad before going out. Both Ray and I were stunned at the news. 'We'll be all right,' I said to Ray later. 'Babies are gifts and we'll get used to the idea. It'll just take time to adjust to the fact that we'll have another little one around before too long.'

It was just as well that Elizabeth had delayed telling me. I had postponed a tutorial, which I should have attended in October because of looking after my Mam, and I had arranged a later date. I had been trying to complete and submit my data presentation and analysis of the questionnaires before going so that my tutor would have time to check it before I arrived. I had found it a lengthy task preparing this piece of work and it would have been even more difficult if I'd had the distraction of Elizabeth's news.

* * *

My reason for using the questionnaires was to collect data about the experiences and particular needs of carers of people with mental illness and whether or not support groups helped in addressing these. I also wished to investigate whether or not a Church-based support group played any part in addressing deeper spiritual needs. The range of questions was multiple in order to cover as many circumstances as possible.

The advantage of fieldwork by use of questionnaires is that it guarantees anonymity in the response as well as assuring that there is no interview bias. It is non-threatening for a carer in that the questionnaire can be completed in the privacy of the home. The questionnaires distributed to the Church-based support group were coded so as to differentiate them on return from those of the secular group. This was to enable me to compare the data received from each group with reference to Church support.

Respondents

Twelve questionnaires had been distributed to the Church-based support group and twenty-six to the secular group. A carers' support worker, recently appointed, had joined the secular group and unfamiliar with the regular attendees, had issued questionnaires to every listed carer from its initiation in 1992, whether or not they currently attended. This may have been an underlying factor in the response to the questionnaires not being higher. Another factor is implied in the comment by a carer who stated that 'over the last couple of years I have been involved in or completed five questionnaires. I know many groups want statistics of our problems, but we need more action'. Also carers who have come through the initial crisis and adapted to some form of acceptance of the situation, may have preferred not to have the initial suffering resurface.

Results

Thirteen of the 26 questionnaires issued to the secular group and 10 of the 12 to the Church-based support group were returned completed.

Opening questions covered

- Gender
- Age
- Length of time as a carer
- Relationship to sufferer

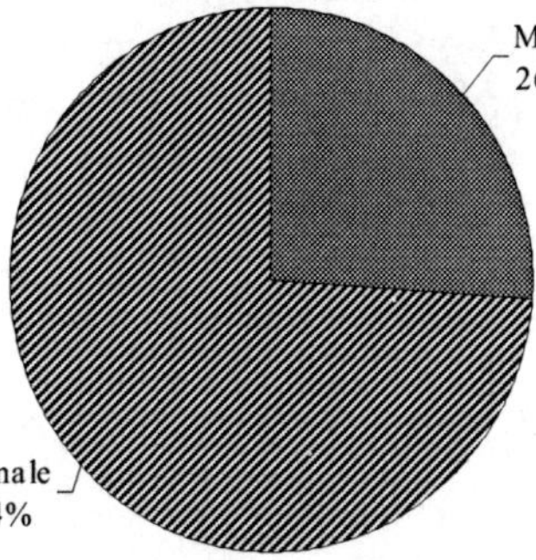

Figure 16.1: Gender of carer

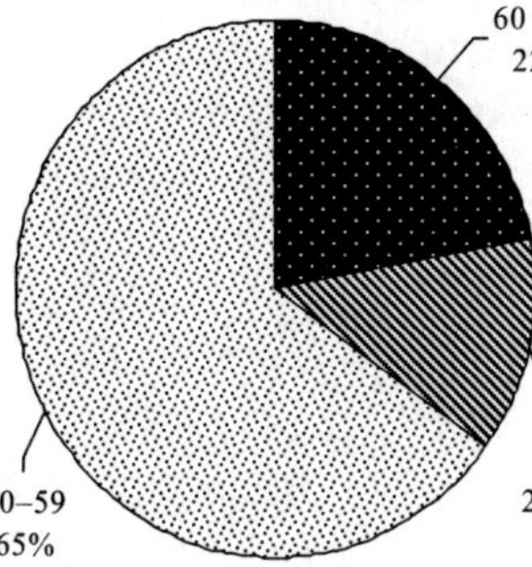

Figure 16.2: Age of carer

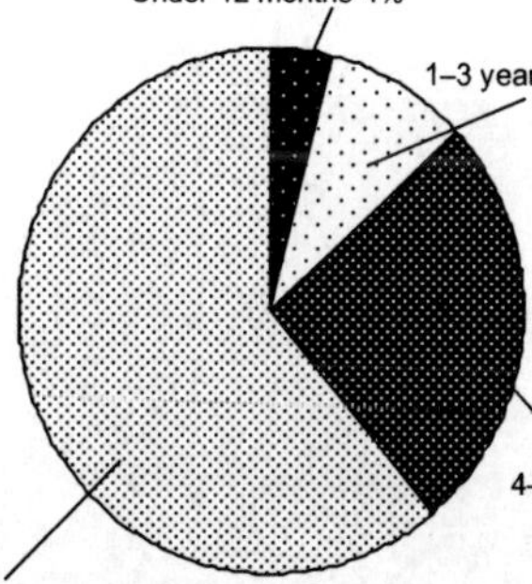

Figure 16.3: Period of time of Caring

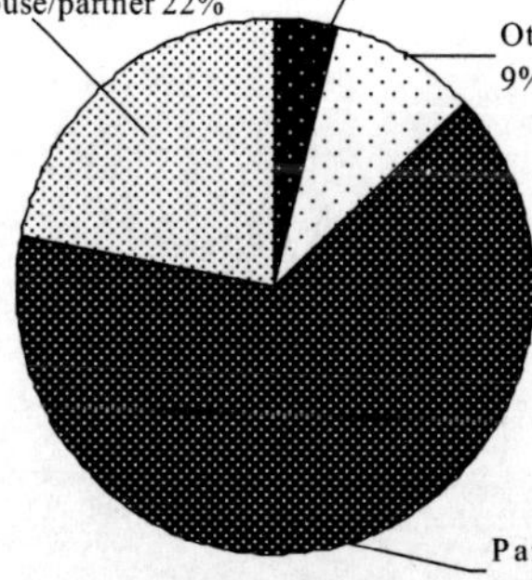

Figure 16.4: Relationship to Sufferer

The conclusion drawn is that a large proportion of the carers are female, middle-aged, and have been caring for an offspring for many years.

Questions on the carer's initial experience and present experience on being accepted and understood as a carer, supported as a carer, and of feeling isolated as a carer with reference to the following:

A	immediate family
B	extended family
C	close friends
D	acquaintances/neighbours
E	colleagues
F	parishioners
G	voluntary community workers
H	clergy
I	medical/professional personnel
J	the sick person's teachers
K	the sick person's colleagues
L	the sick person's friends
M	the sick person's medical/professional personnel

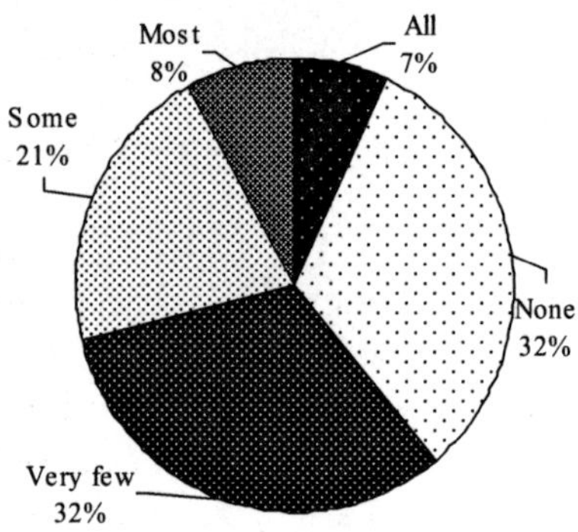

Figure 16.5a: Accepted and understood initally

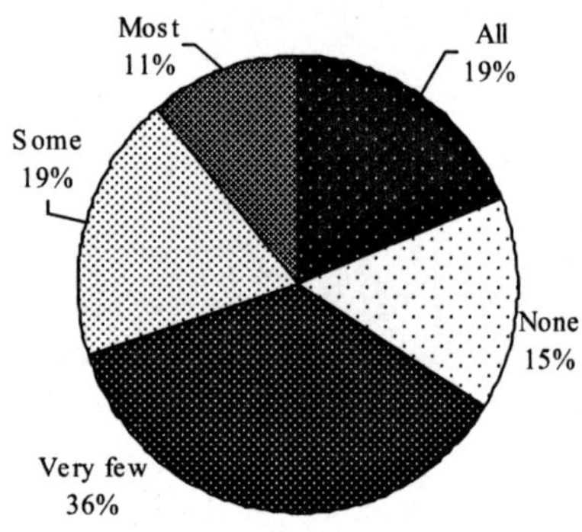

Figure 16.5b: Accepted and understood now

Carers' comments include one who feels the majority of people he mixes with do not want to know about his problems and another that 'in general, being the role of a carer of a person with mental illness in society, you are given very little help and support and understanding compared to a carer of a person with a purely physical illness'. This lack of understanding and appreciation of the role of carers where there is mental illness, was revealed in the literature review (see *Pages119–120; 122; 137–138*).

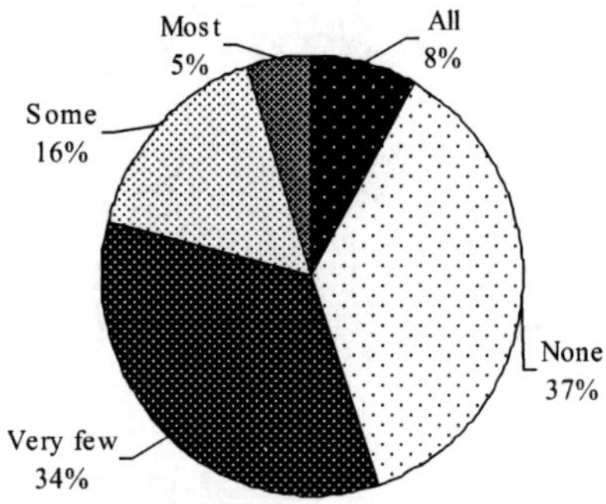

Figure 16.6a: Supported initially

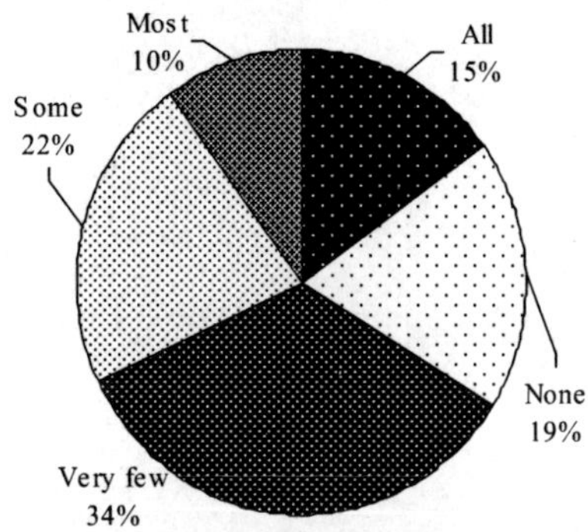

Figure 16.6b: Supported now

Carers' comments include that it is 'difficult to judge opinions as things aren't always black or white'; that 'our local mental health centre is an excellent resource', but another says that 'we need more support in the community for people at home living lives with mental illness'. A carer states that 'my son has been in hospital for quite a while, so now has few friends', and another, that their CPN (community psychiatric nurse) 'moved off after two years and we had nobody to help us'. She adds that nobody asks about their son's behaviour, and professional help is limited to a social worker for their son and 'we feel left on our own to cope', while yet another admits to feeling 'on your own, helpless most of the time'. This research, identifying that carers' needs are neglected, was highlighted earlier (see *Page 119*).

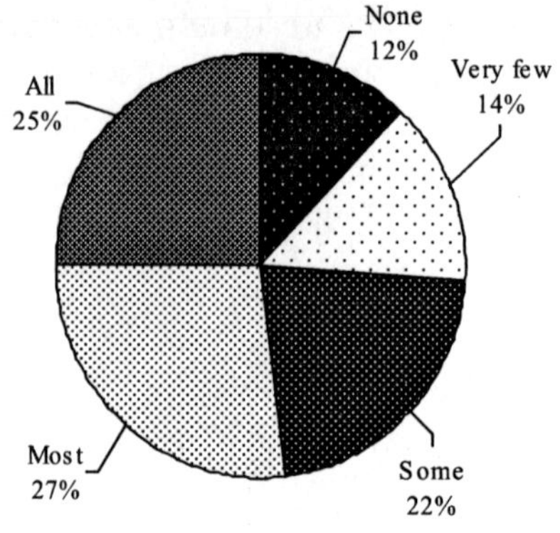

Figure 16.7a: Isolated from initially

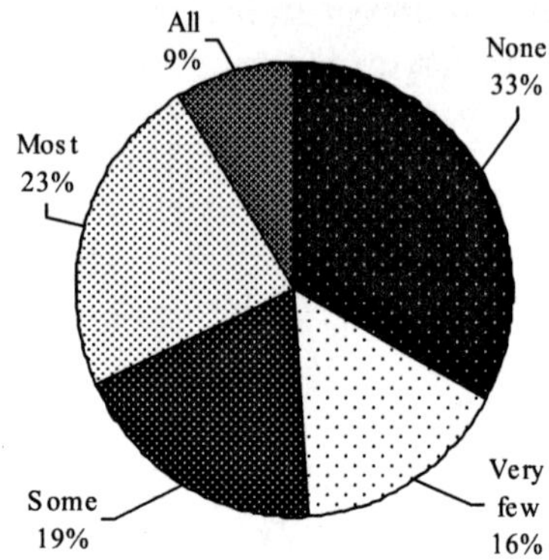

Figure 16.7b: Isolated from now

One carer says she has been disillusioned at the lack of emotional support from her immediate and extended family, but is very grateful to friends for their help. Others comment that 'because, of his age, professional people will not discuss him with me'; and that 'as a rule your situation is rarely mentioned'. These findings, showing that carers experience isolation, identify with those of the literature review (see *Pages 122–123; 136–137*).

Questions relating to Church involvement regarding support

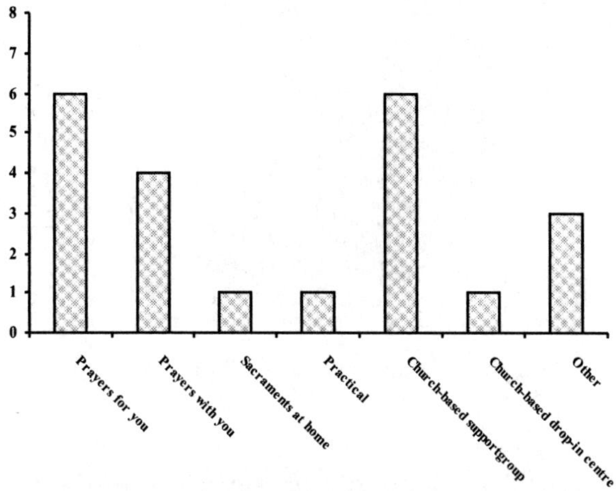

Figure 16.8: Church support: Number respondents out of 8

This graph shows that of the responses from the Scripture-based support group, 80% receive support from the Church leaving 20% who say they do not receive any, which can only be assumed as not receiving support from their specific church community (as the Scripture-based support group is Church support).

Other supports received included being listened to, conversing with others, and receiving advice from a priest who 'was there to turn to'.

Those who responded to the question on how support was initiated said that it was by the Church or friends. Two respondents in the secular group, one of whom requested support, state that they receive Church support, which includes prayer and home visits.

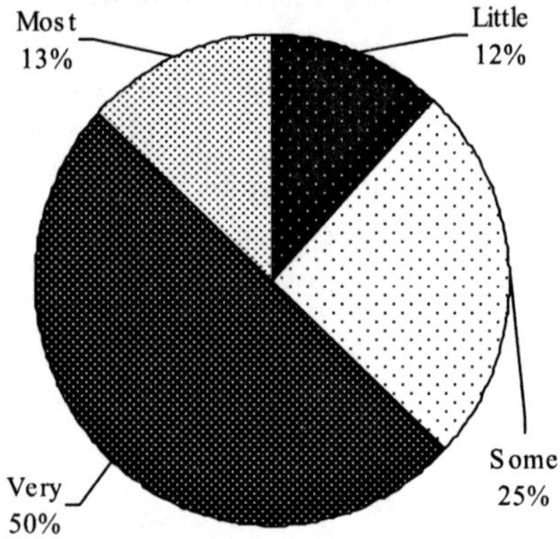

Figure 16.9: Importance of Church support

Reasons given by respondents of the Scripture-based support group for the importance of support are that:

- 'Christ is the Spirit of healing';
- 'I consider myself a devout Catholic, and I try to accept pain and joy as Christ himself did'; and
- 'my church community is part of my life and where I feel I belong. I need their support and understanding'.

A carer says that 'apart from the practical for me, the Church helps greatly with the spiritual side, which these days, society tends to forget about', but another adds that 'it cannot provide total support; only some understanding individuals have done so. It needs to accept mental illness first before helping more'.

Additional comments include one carer not being sure what she wanted and another that 'the meeting place they have provided has been of great help to me, and continues to do so'; that 'people at the church are mostly ignorant about mental illness, so they prefer not to get involved'; and that 'all clergy should have some understanding of mental illness and talk to parishioners about its needs'.

These points agree with the literature review that showed carers need both Church and spiritual support and lack understanding of their needs by the church community (see *Pages 137–138*). They also reinforce the Church's need to assess its missionary role in its involvement in providing care in the community (see *Pages 104–106*). The question also arises as to whether or not the Church is fulfilling its role in supporting families where there is suffering (see *Pages 110–111*). The two respondents of the secular support group say that Church support is very important to them both.

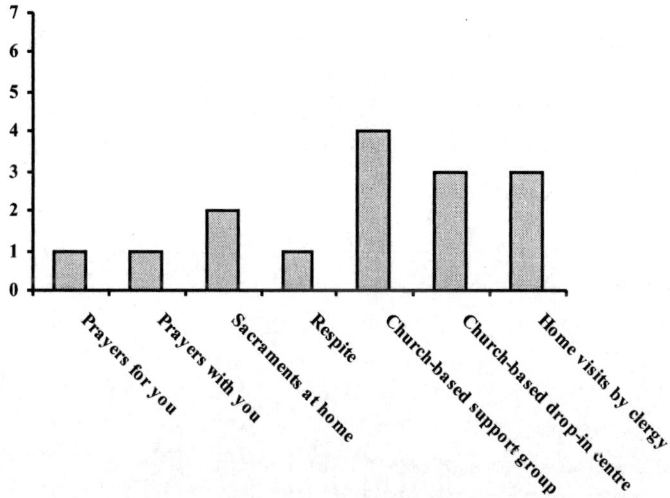

Figure 16.10a: Further Church support wanted: Number of respondents out of 7

Specified support wanted by respondents from the Scripture-based support group is shown in the bar chart above, and in addition 'family counselling and for separate individuals' was requested.

Reasons given for wanting support or further support include showing that 'the Body of the Church cares' and 'I think it would make more people aware of mental distress and break down prejudice over it'. Also that 'when need is there, to be able to go without an appointment to talk' (drop-in centre) and 'for clergy to visit to show value of the sick person and family is as important as in serious physical illness'. Additional comments include a carer saying she feels that a Church-based drop-in centre would be helpful for people in this situation, and another saying that 'when you have nowhere to go for understanding, the Church should have contacts for support day or night. It does not understand how desperate the sufferer and carer are. The Church should be more involved to try and help understand our situation by speaking about mental illness.'

Respondents from the secular support group specify that support wanted includes respite and practical support to make life less stressful together with a Church-based drop-in centre 'as a good place to talk to someone'. One other carer, who had been involved with her church and withdrew because of commitments, says that she has had her faith seriously challenged. She, her husband and son, feel at a low ebb and it is 'sometimes very difficult to keep going'.

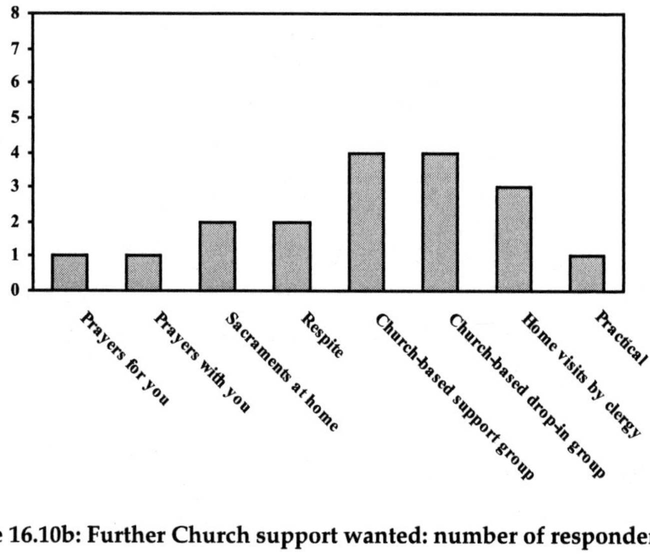

Figure 16.10b: Further Church support wanted: number of respondents out of 8

This bar chart shows the further support wanted from carers of both groups. Carers' needs, both spiritual and pastoral, were expressed in the literature review and suggestions made on how these might be addressed (see *Pages 104–106; 125–127*). The information drawn from the questionnaires shows that these needs have yet to be fulfilled.

Questions relating to involvement in a support group being helpful in the following ways

A	by knowing the Church offers this visible public support
B	by meeting with other carers
C	by being part of a Scripture-based support group
D	by sharing in prayer
E	by relating Scripture to life experiences
F	by addressing your deeper spiritual needs as a carer
G	by the reassurance that the person you care for is accepted
H	in having your feelings of isolation addressed
I	in sharing experiences
J	in sharing feelings
K	by sharing practical advice
L	with information from professionals in this field
M	by sharing different ways of helping the sufferer
N	by having time away from the sufferer
O	in addressing any feelings of shame/stigma through ignorance
P	in addressing any feelings of shame/stigma through fear
Q	in having your role as a carer more understood
R	in feeling more appreciated as a carer
S	in acknowledging that carers fulfil an important role in society
T	to acknowledge that carers are entitled to have their needs addressed

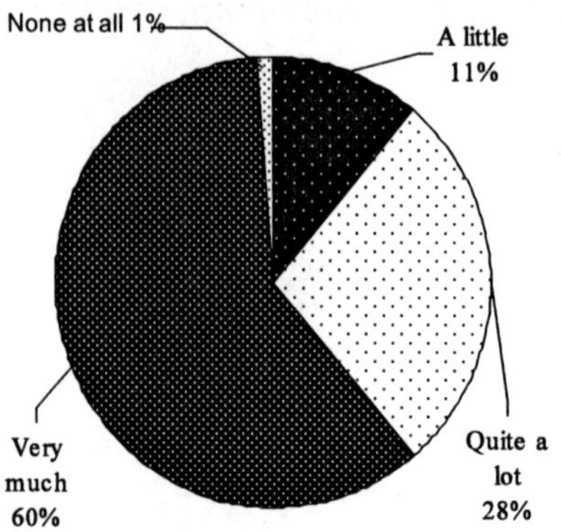

Figure 16.11a: Benefits of support group (Church)

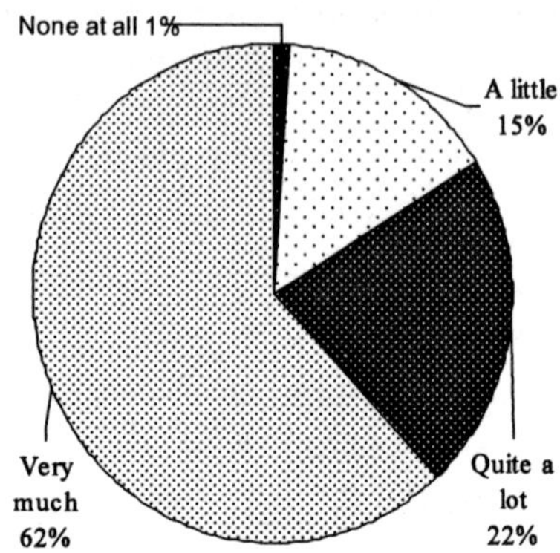

Figure 16.11b: Benefits of support group (Secular)

There is very little difference, as shown in these charts, in degree of benefits experienced by respondents from both groups.

Carers' comments include that 'without the support group I would have felt very vulnerable. It has helped me greatly in as much as I feel a need to attend, not only for myself, but in the hope that I too can be of help to my group. I need the group and quite honestly I would be totally lost without it.' Another says it is 'invaluable' and another two, a 'lifeline'.

Suggestions are that psychiatrists 'should attend these meetings to understand the problems and give advice'; and 'community and Church should provide carers groups and advertise them in newspapers, community centres, council offices etc., so people know of their existence'. Two find difficulty in attending because of family commitments. Another, although acknowledging that a group can help, feels that long-term, it is the carers' responsibility 'to keep loving and helping their dear ones so punished with this dreadful illness and with so little hope for the future'. The importance and value of support groups as revealed in the literature review (see *Pages 124–125; 137–138*) are re-enforced by these findings.

Questions on identifying to what extent respondents thought publicity of support groups achieves the following:

A	raises the importance of carers in society?
B	raises awareness of the need for support?
C	helps educate the public about mental illness?
D	helps in addressing the shame/stigma felt regarding mental illness?
E	helps in addressing the fear of mental illness?
F	helps in the acceptance of mental illness?
G	helps to reassure carers that they are not alone?

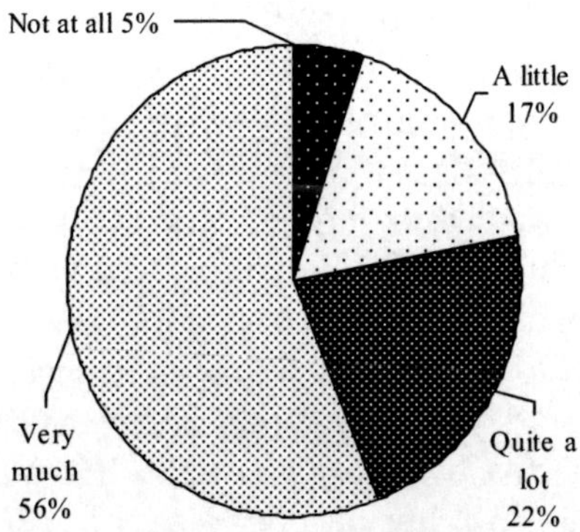

Figure 16.12: Benefits of advertising

Carers' comments include stating that the issue should be 'taken seriously by the Church and society in general'; that 'mental illness is so complex... people are still afraid to speak out. Ignorance is the key factor'; and that much more good publicity is needed. A carer wants anything that will help to educate the general public regarding mental illness and how to handle all aspects. Another wonders why are there very few new members when their group is advertised in surgeries and libraries, and a carer suggests 'more advertising on Radio/TV/newspapers, both locally and nationally to improve attitudes' and that the local paper 'should be less sensational when highlighting' the mental hospital; 'it seems to want to scare people'.

Final comments of carers

A carer states that 'there is a need for much more media exposure of mental illness. Only in this way will society come to terms with its situation. Publicity of the right kind will help. There are too many misleading messages held by society and by opening up, the general public [will] become more caring to the sufferer.' Others comment that 'the general public needs much greater understanding of mental illness. It is generally frightening to them. Also TV programmes don't help much'; and 'we don't see our Royalty visiting mental hospitals, etc. very much and some of them are patrons of mental illness societies' charities'.

A carer hopes that the 'findings can be published to a wider audience or an article produced afterwards and put in [the] local paper or Catholic Voice to highlight the problems faced'. Other comments include that 'carers should be M.O.Td [a reference to cars' annual checks] every six months, i.e. they should be visited by someone to answer their needs'; and 'GPs to be made more aware of mental illness. They should have a back-up service if at all suspicious of problems'. Also that 'there is not enough money to employ well qualified social workers to visit everyone. GPs' knowledge is limited. More counsellors are needed in their surgeries'; and another would like more visits 'from a social worker'. A carer wishes 'the churches had people who reached out of their 'closed' communities to people in need like Jesus did outside the synagogue... I am sure 'they' have a lot to give'; and another carer feels that she cannot ask for Church help because she does not attend.

A carer's prayer 'is for the strength to carry on caring for my son', and one who has had many, many years of caring feels things are much better now for carers; she acknowledges a long history of suffering for all involved 'but we grew'.

A carer concludes that 'only those whose families or close friends have suffered and experienced firsthand the pain of mental illness show understanding. In general, there is, sadly, still a big stigma attached to mental health matters.'

These results show that the stigma, as presented in the literature review (see *Pages 122–123; 136*), is still prevalent in today's society.

* * *

I was very satisfied with this research. Although it was not truly representative, as only carers in the two groups were questioned and others still live in isolation or otherwise, I felt that it gave a lot of insight into what carers feel about society in general and the Church in particular with regards to mental illness. An interesting fact that I discovered during researching was that the secular support group had also been initiated by carers of people with mental illness a year before ours had started. This would seem to signify how isolated these carers had felt and of their great need of understanding, acceptance and support.

My piece of work was finished within my deadline. What a relief. I could now post it and then forget about my dissertation over the Christmas period and concentrate on immediate preparations. I was looking forward to spending more time with my family. Jonathan was coming home for Christmas and Christopher and Stephen would be down from Newcastle.

There is always great hilarity when the lads are staying over as we don't have as many beds since we moved. On one occasion, one of them, when going out, wrote a message for the others left on the mirror in the hall (our means of communication within the family) saying 'I'm having the single bed tonight when I come in.' Another note was added later saying 'no, you are not as I am already in it.'

They come in late at night and have a night cap and watch TV and often fall asleep. The first to wake up claims the single bed. For the second it's the spare mattress on the floor and the last one is left on the settee. But it's all taken in good part. I am looking forward to all the family bantering and what the New Year will bring.

17
OVERVIEW OF SUPPORT AVAILABLE TO CARERS WITHIN THE CATHOLIC CHURCH

Early in 1998 we had yet another surprise. 'Hello, Mam,' said Jacqueline very chirpily when I answered the phone one morning. 'Just to let you know that Benjie's on the way.' It was her way of telling me that she was expecting again. Benjie was going to be Barney's little brother, or so she thought and she was delighted as she wanted two babies close together.

'I think,' I said to Ray, later in the day, 'that you and I will go out and have a drink'. It was just as well that he had his studies to distract him from 'babies'. In October of 1997 in the middle of all the trauma, Ray had begun his MA part-time degree course in archaeology at Durham University. This subject had been his hobby throughout our married life and now, with not working, he was able to pursue his interest with relish.

Another anticipated event for Elizabeth and I was our planned forthcoming pilgrimage to Lourdes. Elizabeth had once told me that she would go back to Lourdes and do all the things she hadn't been able to on our first visit together when she was so ill. Last August we had decided to travel with the Middlesbrough Diocesan Pilgrimage on their next visit to Lourdes this year. Susan was also planning to go with Anne, if Anne was able to travel by plane. Elizabeth still hoped to go even though she would be pregnant, but we had decided to fly instead of travelling by coach and I asked the organisers if the four of us could be together on the flight to Lourdes. When the day arrived we had been allocated places alongside each other. It was wonderful that Anne could travel with us. She had been carried up the steps as she cannot stand or walk and Susan fed her meals to her.

Susan and Anne were staying at the hospital, while Elizabeth and I shared a room in a hotel. Every day we used to go over to the hospital and join Susan and Anne in the planned activities of the day. I had a wonderful pilgrimage. There is something special about helping with a sick person. The four of us were often together with Anne in her wheelchair and Susan pushing it; and Elizabeth, now very pregnant walking on one side with me on the other. Some mornings Elizabeth stayed in bed being too exhausted to go out. She needed a lot of rest. There were times when Anne had to stay at the hospital and rest and Susan and I had time to ourselves. One morning Elizabeth said to me, 'I can pray lying in bed you know, Mam. I'm still making a pilgrimage.' She was right.

I was so pleased that I had written up and posted my dissertation well before making the trip to Lourdes. I had been able to take a complete break after what seemed to me to have been a marathon piece of work. This had included the collating and writing up of the information collected from the interviews with the clergy and doctor. It was a very important part of my dissertation, as I wanted to identify the overall pastoral care of the Church and determine the general support offered to families and carers over a broad spectrum of illness, especially mental illness. I had taped the conversations and Elizabeth had very generously offered to transcribe them for me.

* * *

The interviews of the five selected participants had been conducted with the use of a set of eight questions, which I had designed earlier and had been agreed by my tutor. Advantages of this method is that any questions can be clarified by the interviewee if not clearly understood, before the response is recorded. The list of questions also allows the respondents a certain freedom as the interviewees can give their views in their own time and with the opportunity to give individual responses. Thus, the interview is guided around a framework of selected topics, although still allowing for adaptability. All the interviewees had been given a copy of the questions a few days before being interviewed, so that they would have time to consider their responses.

In your professional role in ministering to people who are ill, to what extent are you involved in supporting their families and/or carers? What importance do you place on this?

The **Vicar General** explained that an administrator in a diocese is responsible for overall pastoral care; that the bishop has a very serious responsibility to make sure that the parish priest is suitable to oversee pastoral care of ill people and this would, logically, include their families and carers. He felt this is particularly important where there are hospitals in parishes.

'It is quite a vital role' said the **hospice chaplain**. He explained that this high degree of importance is shown in the substantial level of support given to families and carers, particularly because of the terminal nature of the sick person's illness.

The **general hospital chaplain** felt that 'it is one of the most important things that I do' and that people with mental illness are 'often the people with their families, in greatest distress'.

The **chaplain to the mental hospital** placed 'great importance in supporting the families of those who are ill' and believed it was very important to be sympathetic to families visiting the mental hospital, as he often found them a little afraid and, sometimes, ashamed. This chaplain is also involved in the local support group for carers/families of people with mental illness held in his parish hall.

The **general practitioner** felt 'it very important' to consider how the person's illness affects their role within the family and he sees ill-health/health presenting in a family situation. With emotional illnesses, he felt 'the impact on the carer tends to be greater'. He stressed that family dynamics were so important that 'it would be very hard to make a full treatment plan' without knowing the whole situation.

What particular needs do you find these families have? Are there specific needs for families of people with mental illness?

The **Vicar General** stated that he would see the first need to be that of understanding on the part of pastoral workers and, therefore, administration would need to try and 'bring about a flow of information and perhaps instruction' to all involved in this work. Where there is mental illness, he sees the families as needing access to 'welcoming and informed pastoral care'.

The **hospice chaplain** said that 'the staff actually view the carers as important in themselves'. His chaplaincy role did not include mental illness, but he added that those families just need someone to talk to, to listen to them; and be given reassurance that God does still exist; that 'there Is still love there'.

The **general hospital chaplain** said that the biggest need for families with someone in hospital is for somebody to spend time with them, 'as much time as I can'; and that they have various needs from the most basic physical requirements 'to needs that are caused by a lack of love'. He admitted that his experience with families of those with mental illness was 'quite limited', but believes they need listening to and often finds himself floundering in 'not knowing what to say to a family struggling with somebody with a mental illness'.

The **mental hospital chaplain** said those families have specific needs because 'mental illness is still stigmatised in our society; that families feel that and they need a great deal of sympathy and empathy'. He has come to realise through the carers support group 'the importance of confidentiality; a relaxed atmosphere where they can meet with other families... share their tears and their pain, their joy and their sorrow and their sometimes lack of hope and sometimes they share their shattered dreams and sometimes just to be nourished by God's Word and to be nourished by a bit of prayer'.

The **general practitioner** stressed needs of education to correct misinformation and of families wanting to talk about their concerns regarding the ill person and how it impinged on them. Needs may include 'physical needs for special aids and adaptations in their houses, or to be led through the maze of the benefit legislation'. He added that 'specific needs are often amplified where there is mental illness', firstly, because there is little information for the carers and also because the person who is 'mentally ill may be so ill that a lot of effort goes into looking after the mentally ill person and it is possible that the carer's own needs can be left behind'.

Comment

In administration, the Vicar General believes that families need access to 'informed pastoral care' where there is mental illness, but the hospice chaplain shows little understanding of their needs in stating that reassurance of God's love and someone to talk to is sufficient. The general hospital chaplain, although acknowledging that these are often the families 'in greatest distress', found difficulty in addressing their needs through lack of experience. The mental hospital chaplain, through his involvement with these families/carers, especially in the support group, shows a deep sensitivity and understanding of their needs. Lack of understanding was highlighted in a previous chapter (see *Pages 104–105*). The general practitioner is concerned with lack of information for these carers and of possible neglect of their needs as discussed earlier (see *Pages119–123; 135–137*).

To what extent does your ministry include support specifically for those families/carers who care for a person who is ill at home/in the community?

The **Vicar General** felt that a key point at administration level would be openness so as to advance in the knowledge of problems, situations and needs of these families/carers, and to see that comments, questions or pleas from individuals are listened to and the response referred back to those involved in their care.

The **hospice chaplain** stated that, in his chaplaincy role, there is little time available for home visits and he directs families to their own parish priests.

The **general hospital chaplain** sees his ministry as being linked with his parish and said that 'the whole community gathered around a church' cares for people in that situation. His ministry includes regular home visits, administering the sacraments and supporting families by listening and giving them time. He gives support to four different community-based carers' groups, for example, Macmillan nurses and clinical psychologists.

The **mental hospital chaplain** added that families/carers of ill people are invited along with the sick to Masses of Anointing and Healing Masses and are sometimes themselves anointed 'to give them strength and support' and are remembered at the weekly Eucharist. The sick in hospital and at home are mentioned in the newsletter to remind the community to pray for them and their carers, and to show that they 'have a very central place in the life and prayer-life of our parish and our weekly Eucharist'.

The **general practitioner** noted that in the community 'specific support to carers is very informal', but 'if there are perceived needs or some special problems,' efforts are made to try and address them. For instance, carers of people with mental illness on several occasions, have been referred to counselling.

What existing services are there available, to your knowledge, which offer support to families of those who are ill, families/carers of people with illness in the community and, specifically, families/carers of people with mental illness?

The **Vicar General** stated that having 'the service of a priest in a parish should automatically imply that there is care for families of those who are ill'. He added that Religious Orders and Parish Sisters have 'taken on a very high profile in families of those who are ill' and that they help in organising and providing respite care and holidays for the sick. Also, a 'whole host of organisations' of lay people are available, plus other local initiatives established that relate to the Handicapped Fellowship. He then added that 'these existing services perhaps could be developed so that the specific needs of those who are suffering from mental illness could be attended to in a more intensive way'.

The **hospice chaplain** felt that in the community 'there is plenty of support for those who are physically ill', that 'Macmillan nurses do a fantastic job' with both the ill person and the family. As for people with mental illness, he stated that all 'I know of is your own organisation... and Mencap, really that is about it, that helps people with mental illness'.

The **general hospital chaplain** found that parish communities 'rally round those who are ill and their families' and that there is plenty of support in the community from lay organisations. He said that there are different kinds of support available for professional carers, particularly at the general hospital, where there are also family units where families support each other and receive professional help. He did not know very much about services available for families and carers of people with mental illness except 'the little support group that you started' and 'organisations like MIND... that would be about it'.

The **mental hospital chaplain** listed much support in the community, including Nazareth House; the hospice; church services; schools in their broadest sense; nurses giving free time to take the sick to Lourdes; and the Catholic Handicapped Fellowship, which, he said, have a whole network of support including worshipping together, a youth club, holidays organised and day trips and respite care offered by the religious. He felt that 'the Church has been lacking in care for the families of people with mental illness', but feels that there is effort being made to raise awareness in the diocese 'of this particular deficiency'. He knows that priests, some better than others, provide support within the parishes on an individual basis, and that 'we have this monthly meeting in our parish hall here, which is an invitation to people across the town and across the region to come along. It is publicly advertised'. He added that, recently, attempts have been made to have barbecues and bingo afternoons in order to 'make the carers and families of people with mental illness part of our community by reaching out to them'.

The **general practitioner** stated that 'existing services are not spread as wide as we would like to see them'. He said that emotional support is given in hospital wards alongside the support of the hospital chaplain and sometimes more formal counselling is available, but that much greater numbers in the community make the support more patchy. He feels that Macmillan nurses and Marie Curie nurses are the exception rather than the rule and 'for this reason families have formed self-help groups'. A self-help group, he said, 'is a marvellous thing and it shows people are trying to improve things for themselves'. He added that 'in the specific area of families and carers of people with mental illness, we are fortunate locally to have a group that meets quite informally on a regular basis for carers to come and talk about their feelings where people can support each other'. He knows it is advertised in local general practitioners' surgeries and local churches and concluded that, as it is denominational, he has been very happy to recommend it to carers who are feeling the strain. Counselling is available, he added, for carers at his practice even for patients not on their lists although 'not as widespread as I would like to see it'.

Comment

These findings show that, in comparison with help in other areas, support where there is mental illness appears to be minimal. The only Church support known to two chaplains was the carers' support group. The Vicar General speaks of openness to advance in the knowledge of needs and suggests that existing services perhaps could be developed so that specific needs of those who are suffering mental illness (and presumably their families/carers) could be supported in a more intensive way. The hospice chaplain showed a lack of knowledge of mental illness by referring to Mencap as a resource because it is for those with learning difficulties. The mental health chaplain, who is involved with these families, acknowledges a deficiency in the Church's pastoral care where there is mental illness which raises questions regarding the Church fulfilling its role as detailed earlier (see *Pages 110–114*).

How are these services funded, structured and administered?

The **Vicar General** reported that there is a looseness about funding, structuring and administration and 'maybe that such things need to be looked at'. Parish activity depends on how the priest sees needs and the diocese is structured and administered as part of the general activity of the diocese/parish.

The **hospice chaplain** thought the hospice funding was voluntary from people's generosity. He said that the priest 'does it for a minimal wage' and the lay people do it for nothing at all. Administration, he felt, is not necessary as the response is to the Gospel fulfilling Christ's command of looking after 'those more vulnerable and those in more need than ourselves.

The **general hospital chaplain** stated that MIND is a national service with moneys from the lottery and a little from the council. He said that everything else is all charity-based work, and trying to give any kind of structure to it would be almost impossible.

Neither the **hospice chaplain** nor the **mental hospital chaplain** knew how services of the state were funded, but the **mental hospital chaplain** felt that the Church has to work in partnership with the state and local services. He knows that the bishop is generous in quiet ways but feels, from the Church point of view, there is a deficiency. He describes the endless voluntary support in the community as 'self-generating.'

In terms of service in the hospitals, the **general practitioner** stated that the professionals find time in their busy schedules, which is, therefore, funded through their salaries, but generally in a haphazard way. Macmillan nurses are a mixture of state funding and charitable donations. As far as carers of those with mental illness, 'the input from the state to my knowledge is nil and in many ways that is reprehensible'. He stated that people surrounded by illness 'themselves have needs and yet in planning services, their needs seem to be taking a back seat'.

How well do you think that the state's available existing services for carers of people suffering a mental illness support those carers?

Neither the **Vicar General** nor the **hospice chaplain** knew of any. The **Vicar General** felt that from the reports through the press and problems thrown up as a consequence of the Community Care Act 'and the generally disastrous cases that bring this situation into focus, it would seem that the state's existing services for carers of people suffering from mental illness leave something to be desired'.

The **general hospital chaplain** thought that 'professional carers in the plural are catered for quite well' and commented that 'at the end of the day it is a job and they can walk away.' He thought there were some services for carers of family members, but 'I am sure that it could be a lot better than it already is'.

The **mental hospital chaplain** said that what there was in the hospital was voluntary and usually set up by willing staff, who also took patients on day trips, but as for the carers, he felt services were lacking. He knew of a community-based advocacy project started this year and of a day care centre giving respite and also a hostel.

The **general practitioner** stated that the state 'does a miserable job in attempting to support carers' and that 'available existing services appear to largely exclude carers'. He is aware of a support group at the local mental health day facility, again initiated by carers. Local authorities are now starting to consider carers, but 'it is at the embryonic stage and I believe relatively modern'.

Comment

The Vicar General suggests that state services for carers of people with mental illness are deficient. The hospice chaplain had no knowledge of them. The general hospital chaplain commented that professional carers are catered for quite well and 'at the end of the day can walk away'. He was unsure about services for family carers, but feels that there is room for improvement. Both the mental hospital chaplain and the general practitioner feel that the state's provision is inadequate, reflecting the neglect of community care cited in the literature review (see *Page 120*).

If services are in any way inadequate, does the Church play a vital role in adding to these services? How well do you feel the Church is currently fulfilling its preferential option for the poor, sick and other special needs groups in the support it offers to carers of people suffering a mental illness?

The **Vicar General** commented that 'the Church must play a vital role in any activity that is related to the Gospel values that we stand for', but he wondered whether it does, in adding to these services. He felt that 'there is probably an overwhelming regard for education in its broadest sense' and 'the Church in other areas of social need is perhaps not as sufficient as it might be'.

The **hospice chaplain** stated that 'the Church has always played a vital role' in adding to state services and that 'I felt myself, very strange that you put all this stress on the carers of mental illness because I don't differentiate between the people I am visiting'. He states that clergy have so many demands made on their time that they 'cannot formulate a structured response to all the people with different needs', and neither does he feel the Church particularly picks out any specific group. He feels that help is given where it is needed 'adequately or inadequately, but if there is no training, there is nothing else that we can do'. He added that it is the people involved 'that can tell the Church what needs to be done'. He believes it is they who should be leading forward and asking for whatever support the Church can give rather than 'the Church hierarchy, which is what I feel you mean by the Church'. He said that we are all Church and 'if we do not play our own part properly, then virtually somebody is going to suffer'.

The **general hospital chaplain** said that the Church does play a vital role in adding to these services, but if he was being asked if the Church is fulfilling Gospel values that it preaches in offering support to these carers, then his response was that there are some great individuals 'who are as Christ-like as it is possible to be', but sadly some 'don't feel able or they don't recognise the needs of somebody in that situation'.

The **mental hospital chaplain** believes that the Church has to play a vital role in adding to these services because he feels that state care is inadequate. He stressed that Our Lord ministered to the sick very much on a one to one and 'always found time' and was always 'recognising the dignity of that person' and added that the Church has to recognise that these people have their dignity. This chaplain feels that 'the Church is waking up and awareness is being raised that our support is inadequate' and suggests home-visiting where there is mental illness. He also proposes that clergy be trained more adequately 'to help them to deal with this type of ministry'; that maybe in the seminary, part of their training should be for ministering to people with mental illness and as 'everybody is doing a lot of self-examination' as we approach this millennium, that 'maybe that is one of the ways that the Church again can rediscover its preferential option for the poor and the sick, and support the people and families of those with mental illness'.

The **general practitioner** said that he feels strongly that 'the Church does have a preferential option for treating special needs groups in our community'. He suggests there may be a problem 'that perhaps with mental health being the Cinderella subject there is a lot more attractiveness in sending (money) to a third world where people are starving than in supporting carers'. He stated that 'when you consider the amount that the Church spends on buildings, education and other structures within the community, which are vital and important, it doesn't take too much imagination to see how much a little bit of money can do in providing some key workers for supporting carers'.

Comment

The Vicar General doubts whether the Church is playing a vital role in the area of mental illness and sees a possible need for improvement in areas of social need. The hospice chaplain implies a lack of training and also believes that the people involved ought to lead. The general hospital chaplain expresses the inadequacy of some personnel and the mental hospital chaplain acknowledges inadequate support and recommends more competent training for clergy. The general practitioner is concerned that mental illness is a Cinderella area with regard to resources and that this needs addressing by the Church. This research reflects what was said in earlier chapters about lack of Church support (see *Pages 104–106; 125–126; 138*).

Do you have any further comment you would like to make regarding what you see as the Church's responsibility in supporting carers in general, and specifically carers of people suffering a mental illness?

The **Vicar General** began by stating that 'you, Edna, have made me a lot more aware of this whole question than I had been and probably ever would be. So I would commend that'. He then added that this is 'probably reflecting a need, within the life of the Church in general to bring the issue sharply into focus in a way that would be accepted by both lay people and clergy, so that it becomes very much highlighted'. He stated that pastoral care of carers has gone on for a long time, but suggested that now these needs be presented in a wholesome way so that people can take this on board 'and respond to it rather than see it as an isolated and specialist activity'.

The **hospice chaplain** again stated that there is no need 'to specify one particular group' as the Church has a responsibility to look after everybody. He is aware that 'some people feel marginalised and ostracised by the Church' but thinks 'that a lot of the time it is not the Church's fault'. He feels the Church wants to help, but that it does not have the resources nor the capacity to look after those who need most help. He is aware that mental illness 'is still seen by society at large as having a stigma' and feels the response to it 'on the part of the officials, is quite often one of fear rather than acceptance'. He concluded that, in caring for physically ill and mentally ill people, 'there is a great difference I think'.

The **general hospital chaplain** concluded that when talking about the Church's responsibility, 'we have to be very careful about how we define the Church' as 'priests on the whole are greatly over-stretched'. He added that great demands are made on priests' time and he has found it difficult to do all that is expected of him with 'very little specialised training'.

The **mental hospital chaplain** said that bridges need to be built 'and we have got to educate people more about mental illness to break down prejudice and stigma' as there is always going to be mental illness in our communities, and the Church's responsibility is to have 'a special sensitivity, a special welcome' to these families.

The **general practitioner** 'would like to see more done for people caring for someone suffering from a mental illness.' He felt that the Church's role in this 'needs to be expanded, and can only be, if some resources are put towards it'. He said that 'the vast majority of people with mental health problems are being looked after by concerned carers, usually of their own family'. Where a specific religion is concerned he feels that 'they need emotional as well as practical support from the Church'. He concluded that the needs of carers 'have to be acknowledged first and helped second' and that 'the Church has to do more' than just give verbal sympathy.

Comment

The Vicar General acknowledges to only recently becoming much more aware of this area of pastoral need. The hospice chaplain believes that there is no need to specify one particular group, but this is questionable given the Church's teaching in an earlier chapter (see *Pages 113–114*). The general practitioner wants carers' needs acknowledged and then addressed by the Church. In this research regarding mental illness, the Church acknowledges prejudice, stigma and fear; a need for education and training of clergy; and notes a shortage of Church resources. It would appear these factors need addressing in order to implement what the Vicar General describes as bringing the issue 'sharply into focus'.

* * *

I had found the responses very enlightening especially the differences in the understanding of carers' sufferings and their needs. The interviewees had, I felt, been very open and honest in their replies, which helped greatly in building a representative picture of the degree of importance placed on caring, especially of someone with a mental illness. I was looking forward to drawing the whole picture together.

On our return from Lourdes, Elizabeth started going to Mass every Sunday evening in her parish church. She had made her peace with God. One Sunday, three weeks later, she came home around teatime. 'You know, Mam, it's quite lonely on my own at church. I don't know anyone.' 'Elizabeth,' I said, 'I would willingly come with you, but I didn't like to interfere. I didn't think you'd want me to come with you.'

'Well I would actually, Mam.' I was pleased to go with her and we went each week right up to her having her baby. While on maternity leave, she spent a lot of time with me. Jacqueline and Elizabeth enjoyed sharing the ups and downs of pregnancy, but as Elizabeth's expected date grew closer, I became more and more anxious, even though I was looking forward very much to her baby's arrival. Would all go well?

18
FINDINGS, CONCLUSIONS AND RECOMMENDATIONS

The last weeks before a baby arrives seem exceedingly long. Elizabeth was getting very heavy and wondering if the baby would come early. I think I lived her aches and pains each day with her as she waited anxiously for the baby's arrival. We saw a lot of Heather, Stephanie's baby girl, who was now beginning to talk and when asked where Elizabeth's baby was, would pat Elizabeth's tummy and say, 'baby.' Barnaby was crawling and needed constant watching when we minded him. Aware that my dissertation was now being examined, I looked back over my concluding chapter, wondering if it was satisfactory.

I looked at the major points concerning caring, especially where there is mental illness and put them into categories. I read through all my chapters and marked the pieces relevant to these and collated them. The following is a summary of the whole piece of work.

* * *

Scope of literature

Perrin *et al* (1990) find that literature on carers tends to concentrate on carers of people needing physical support and that literature on families caring for people diagnosed with a mental illness has been neglected. They also find that literature in the psychiatric and psychological fields rarely looks at carers in their own right. Church teaching does not specifically mention carers in its teaching on pastoral care, but does include a number of teachings on the alleviation of all kinds of human needs (AA 8). The literature on carers and Church support is minimal. The general practitioner agrees that 'there is little information' either on, or for carers of people with mental illness.

Care in the Community

Wainright (1997) states that the burden of care in the community rests more heavily on carers of people with mental illness than ever before and Hogman and Pearson (1995) that their needs are neglected. Atkinson and Coia (1995) state that there is little evidence of a caring community and suggest that, in reality, care in the community is the family. The Church teaches that the joy and hope, the grief and anguish of people, especially those afflicted in any way, are the joy and hope, the grief and anguish of the followers of Christ (GS 1). The Church teaches in *The International Year of Disabled Persons* that Christians need to stand alongside organisations to foster support and increase initiatives to help alleviate suffering. Burton-Jones (1992) suggests that the potential for churches in providing support to vulnerable people is at its greatest in this era and is a consequence of the Care in the Community Act (1990). She feels that the Church will need to assess to what extent it should become formally involved in providing care and perhaps consider working in partnership with other concerned groups. The Jubilee Centre (1990) believes the local church could play a significant role in meeting needs not met by statutory bodies.

My own fieldwork found agreement that state services are lacking. The general practitioner adds that local authorities are starting to consider carers but 'it is at the embryonic stage and I believe relatively modern' and the mental hospital chaplain feels that the Church has to work in partnership with the state and local services. Carers, themselves, feel totally unsupported by a fifth of those they are in contact with, which includes family, friends, state services and Church, and from over a third they feel very little support. They feel more supported than at the initial stages of their caring role, but still only feel fully supported by a small number. One carer describes it as feeling 'on your own, helpless most of the time' and another that 'we feel left on our own to cope'.

The information gathered from my interviews shows that the Church offers an abundance of support to families and carers where there is illness in general, and the general practitioner stresses that family dynamics are so important that 'it would be very hard to make a full treatment plan' without knowing the full situation. Where there is mental illness, the Vicar General suggests that perhaps existing services be developed so that those suffering mental illness (and presumably their families and carers) 'could be attended to in a more intensive way' because, while there is an overwhelming regard for education in its broadest sense, 'the Church in other areas of social need is perhaps not as sufficient as it might be'. Church support for these carers is minimal, two chaplains being aware of the Church-based support group as the only service on offer. The mental hospital chaplain feels 'it is true to say that the Church has been lacking in care for the families of people with mental illness' but that effort is being made to raise awareness 'of this deficiency'.

Funding

Twigg and Atkin (1994: 114) found that carers of people with mental illness, in terms of priority for local authority funding, 'have been pushed to the back of the queue'. Hogman and Pearson (1995) found the majority of studies investigating financial situations of carers discovered that they have difficulties with regard to finances, which are directly related to having a member of the family suffering a mental illness, and that respite care, which was wanted by three-quarters of carers in their survey, would clearly benefit carers financially as well as health wise. Chiu (1988) is also aware that carers are obliged to adapt to limited resources.

The Vicar General feels that Church funding, structuring and administering may need to be looked at, but the hospice chaplain believes administration of funding is not necessary as the response is to the Gospel in looking after 'those more vulnerable than ourselves'. The hospital chaplain sees funding as charity-based and, therefore, 'trying to give any kind of structure to it would be almost impossible'. The general practitioner agrees, in relation to mental illness, that people surrounded by illness have needs 'and yet in planning services their needs seem to be taking a back seat'. He feels, with reference to the Church, that perhaps as mental health is a Cinderella area, it is a less attractive option for financial support, and yet a little financial help to providing means of support for carers would be money well spent. He believes that the Church's role in supporting carers of people with mental illness needs to be expanded and can only be 'if some resources are put towards it'.

Stress and isolation

Burton-Jones (1992) found that the carer undergoes much distress through the attitude of the sufferer because of personality changes, especially where there is mental illness. McCann (1995) found that stress is heightened because responsibility tends to fall consistently on one individual in the family, and Atkinson and Coia (1995) feel this to be particularly true where there is mental illness. McCann states that carers in the home have held the Cinderella position within the whole field of caring and families largely go unnoticed.

Moate and Enoch (1990) state that there are considerable levels of disruption to family life where there is mental illness, which Twigg and Atkin (1994) find, includes marriage ties being weakened. Perrin *et al* (1990) find that a person with mental illness can become increasingly demanding of their family, which can act as a severe restraint on the carer's life, leading to the carer's social life being severely restricted. This, Moate and Enoch say, leads to isolation from the rest of the world and carers having feelings of helplessness and hopelessness. Hogman and Pearson (1995) find this isolation is felt, even from family and friends. The Jubilee Centre (1990) tells of a carer who speaks of this despair and isolation and Edginton (1993) of one crying every day and eventually trying to commit suicide.

The Church teaches that if one member of Christ's body suffers, then all suffer and, consequently, help given for the relief of human want should be held in high esteem (HD 33). The general hospital chaplain agrees that people with mental illness are 'often the people with their families in greatest distress' and the general practitioner also agrees that, with emotional illnesses, 'the impact on the carer tends to be greater'.

Carers, themselves, feel some degree of isolation from two-thirds of people and mostly isolated from almost a quarter. A carer states that 'you are given very little help, support and understanding compared to a carer of a person with a purely physical illness'.

Stigma, publicity and education

Twigg and Atkin (1994) state that, in general, carers feel they have to cope with a world that does not want to understand their situation. Burton-Jones (1992) feels the lack of understanding is because empathy for the carer can be very painful and carers are mostly invisible. Burningham (1989) sees an outcome of this lack of understanding is the likelihood of carers seeing their situation as something of which to be ashamed. Moate and Enoch (1990) found that ignorance and fear are two powerful forces that have prevented the advancement of care and Stobbart (1996) states that some carers avoid contact with friends and neighbours because of shame, and fear of stigma. Atkinson and Coia (1995) say that mental illness has always been stigmatised, which has come about and still does from a largely ill-informed public. Wallace (1996) feels that media publicity generates stigma and what is needed is a campaign for better help for the sufferer and understanding for families. Moate and Enoch tell of a carer who was filled with the horror of the word 'schizophrenia' before diagnosis.

The Church teaches in *The International Year of Disabled Persons* that those responsible for planning programmes in social care and integration of disabled people should make the family the starting point, as families need to be given great understanding and sympathy to help prevent feelings of isolation and rejection. It adds that people do not want to face negative aspects of life, but this gives rise to exclusion and discrimination and, therefore, this tendency must be countered by education. Pope John Paul II says that love goes beyond those of the same faith and knows how to discover the face of Christ 'in each individual, especially the weak and those who suffer' (FC 64). The Southwark Diocesan Board (1994) state that fear, rejection, and expressions of misunderstanding may all be experienced by the carer of someone with mental illness from in the community, including their church. Ledger (1992) suggests church members becoming actively involved in voluntary bodies so that the Christian

Church 'can help break down the social stigma attached to disability and mental illness and thus support carers'.

In this current piece of research, the Vicar General agrees that pastoral workers need understanding; that administration needs to 'bring about a flow of information and perhaps instruction' and 'openness so as to advance in knowledge of problems, situations and needs'. He adds that, where there is mental illness, families need access to 'informed pastoral care' and there is probably a need to bring the issue 'sharply into focus'.

The hospice chaplain, by suggesting Mencap as a support for people with mental illness, demonstrates his lack of knowledge of mental illness because Mencap is an organisation for people with learning difficulties. He disagrees with the need 'to specify any particular need' because the Church has a responsibility to look after everybody, but agrees that mental illness 'is still seen by society at large as having a stigma' and that response to it 'on the part of the officials, is quite often one of fear rather than acceptance'.

The chaplain to the mental hospital agrees that families of a sufferer of a mental illness are a little fearful and ashamed sometimes, that 'mental illness is still stigmatised in our society'. He agrees with the need for education and proposes that clergy be trained more adequately 'to help them deal with this type of ministry'.

The information gathered from the questionnaires reveals that, initially, carers experienced a total lack of understanding from almost a third of people, and although the number of those who now fully appreciate their role has trebled, it is still barely a fifth of the people with whom they are in contact. Carers agreed that 'people at church are mostly ignorant about mental illness'. A carer feels that 'all clergy should have some understanding of mental illness and talk to parishioners about it' as does another who says that 'the Church should be more involved to try and help understand our situation by speaking about mental illness'. A carer feels that more Church support would 'make more people aware of mental distress and break down prejudice' and another agrees that 'people are still afraid to speak out. Ignorance is the key factor'. They see that anything beneficial to educating the general public is needed, plus more advertising through the press, both locally and nationally to improve attitudes.

Support groups

McCann (1995) found that support groups are particularly helpful because of the support carers can give to each other and Kupiers *et al* (1989) state that they are cost-effective support for carers. Atkinson and Coia (1995) found that they are educational for the participants, are also aimed at the general public to heighten awareness of carers' problems, and reduce stigma. Carson (1992) discovered that they help in overcoming the feelings of stigma and shame and McCann found they help prevent feelings of isolation and provide a social outlet. Stobbart (1996) found that they were a lifeline to many. Wainright (1997) discovered that some carers did not wish to meet with others similarly situated, as they felt barely able to cope with their own family. Hogman and Pearson (1995) found that carers' contact with their peer group is a vital part of community care and that service providers and purchasers ought to build up relationships with carer groups.

The Church teaches in *The International Year of Disabled Persons* that professionals and volunteers who give themselves to the service of the disabled should 'learn to dialogue with the parents and families' and also that 'a prudent pastoral commitment, modelled on Our Lord, is called for in families who find themselves in difficult situations' (FC 77). Oglesby (1984) suggests that keeping the Law of Christ is carrying each others burdens and sees this as the People of God journeying together holding hands. Ledger (1992) feels that the greatest aspect of Jesus' ministry was his willingness to enter into the human situation and, similarly, there is need to give time and energy to carers to allow them the freedom to express their feelings. The Jubilee Centre (1990) suggests that introducing Christian carers to one another is a way of supporting them, and so, too, is organising drop-in coffee mornings to help counteract feelings of isolation. The Newcastle Diocesan Board (1996) suggests the facilitating of self-help groups and the establishing of Church-based support groups, as they are lifelines to many.

The hospice chaplain believes that clergy have many demands made on them and that it should be the people involved who should be leading forward and organising groups, and not leaving it to the Church hierarchy who have not always had training. The general hospital chaplain states that some do not feel able to help and some do not recognise the needs of these carers. The mental hospital chaplain agrees on the value and importance of Church-based support groups for carers of people with mental illness from his experience of the local one. The general practitioner also agrees a self-help group is 'a marvellous thing' and adds that 'we are fortunate locally to have a group where people can support each other'.

The carers agree on the value of support groups, with well over half finding them very beneficial and over a quarter finding quite a lot of support from them. Carers say how helpful they have been, that 'I would be totally lost without it'; it is 'invaluable'; and a 'lifeline'.

Spiritual support

Swinton and Kettles (1997) feel that an individual needs to be respected as a person holistically because when individuals' spirituality is taken into account, they are seen as persons and not as problems. Pratt *et al* (referred to by Atkinson and Coia, 1995) name spiritual support as one of two aids associated with significantly less carer burden. McCann (1995) believes that 'everyone has profound spiritual needs', which, lying below the surface of the carer's consciousness, will inevitably surface and maybe do so with great force. McCann states that spiritual pain is a profound reality that, 'may be the pain that requires most attention and help,' and adds that it concerns the depths of what it means to be human. Moate and Enoch (1990) feel there must be particular concern about lack of support by Christian Churches where there is mental illness. Ledger (1992) tells of a carer who longed for someone to show love and concern for him and of another who believes that emotional, spiritual and practical support are so important and suggests that the Church can help in encouragement, prayer and practical help.

The Church teaches that it is the duty of those who help the sick to attend to both physical and spiritual needs, as it was Christ's intention 'that the whole person should be their concern and that they should offer both physical relief and spiritual comfort' (HD 4) because he was concerned about both (HD 5); and that a person should be considered, whole and entire (GS 3). In *The International Year of Disabled Persons*, the Church teaches that many people undergo stress and shock that disturb their psychic and interior life, and it is important that the health of the spirit is fostered so that a person is not damaged in his deeper needs.

Chiu (1988) feels that it is not possible to separate spiritual life from a person's psychological life and there is a need for an integrated understanding of what is a human being's psychological development coupled with spiritual formation. Burton-Jones (1992) states that caring generates intense spiritual yearnings, which the Church, in its pastoral care, must address, and suggests enabling a carer to make a retreat in order to recharge physical, spiritual and emotional batteries. The Southwark Diocesan Board (1994) reports the Bishop of Woolwich saying that bearing some of this pain must be at the heart of Christian ministry.

In the case of the current findings, the Vicar General agrees that the bishop has a very serious responsibility to make sure the parish priest is suitable to oversee pastoral care of ill people, their families and carers. He adds that pastoral care of carers has gone on for a long time, but suggests that now this particular need be presented in a wholesome way, so that people can take it on board and respond rather than see it as an isolated and specialist activity. All three chaplains place great importance on the role of ministering to families and carers of ill people. The hospice chaplain feels that carers of people with mental illness just need someone 'to listen to them' and reassurance that God still does exist. The general hospital chaplain has had little experience of these carers, but feels they need listening to. The researcher found these comments not wholly in agreement with findings in the literature review, unlike the mental hospital chaplain's views, as he has come to understand, particularly through the support group, the depth of their needs, and that includes spiritual nourishment. He also suggests home visiting where there is mental illness.

I found that, of the carers of the Church-based support group, almost all state that they are receiving support from the Church, which is important to them. Three quarters mention the support group from which both Church and spiritual support received is much appreciated. Seven of the ten respondents would like more support from the Church as would one from the secular group. Half of these would like a Church-based drop-in centre and half would like a Church-based support group with almost a third wanting home visits from a priest/minister. A carer says that the Church helps greatly with the spiritual side, which society tends to forget about, but another stated that it cannot provide total support because it needs to accept mental illness first before helping more. One finds the meeting place they have provided has been of great help. One, who was involved with Church, had to withdraw and finds her faith seriously challenged. A home visit by clergy was wanted to show that value of the sick person and family is as important as in serious physical illness. Two respondents of the secular group receive Church support of prayer and home visits and this is very important to them.

Conclusions

Twigg and Atkin (1994) state that carers tend to be neglected and McCann (1995) says that there is need for recognition and status, for education and support, of community-based facilities and respite care. Hogman and Pearson (1995) state that the carers have now become the silent partners in community care. I believe that they have deep spiritual needs and Ledger (1992) says that the only really lasting hope for carers is in Jesus Christ. The Church teaches that wherever people are racked by misfortune or illness, they should be comforted with devoted care and given support that will relieve their needs, and today these works of charity have become much more urgent. Charitable action should reach all needs (AA 8). Pope John Paul II admonishes that priests and deacons 'must support the family in its difficulties and sufferings' (FC 73). Ledger concludes that, were Jesus here today in person, he would be aware of carers' deep emotional and spiritual needs and asks that the Holy Spirit be allowed to bring love, comfort and support to carers.

In interview, the Vicar General, having been made aware of this whole issue of carers of people with mental illness very recently, agrees that it is probably a need within the life of the Church to have the issue highlighted in a way that would be accepted by both people and clergy. The hospice chaplain also agrees that some people feel marginalised and ostracised by the

Church, but disagrees that it is just the Church's fault as the Church wants to help, but has neither the resources, nor the capacity to look after those who need most help. He acknowledges that there is a great deal of difference between caring for physically and mentally ill people. The hospital chaplain states that it is necessary to be careful when defining what is meant by 'Church' and that great demands are made on priests with very little specialised training. The mental hospital chaplain points out that, as there is always going to be mental illness in communities, the Church's responsibility is to have a special sensitivity, and a special welcome to these families. He also agrees that bridges need to be built and people have to be educated more about mental illness to break down prejudice and stigma.

The general practitioner also agrees that the vast majority of people with mental health problems are being looked after by concerned carers, usually one of their family, and that he would like to see more done for carers of people with mental illness. He feels that, where a specific religion is concerned, they need emotional as well as practical support from the Church, but their needs have to be acknowledged first and helped second. He concludes that the Church has to do more than give verbal sympathy.

Carers conclude that mental illness needs much more media exposure and good publicity, for only in this way will society come to terms with its situation. It is generally frightening to them and TV does not help much. Carers feel that too many misleading images are held by society and by opening this up, the general public, who need much greater understanding of mental illness, will become more caring to the sufferer. A carer comments that members of the Royal family are not often seen visiting mental hospitals, and yet some are patrons of mental illness societies' charities. Another hopes that these findings can be published to a wider audience, or an article produced and published in the local paper or Catholic Voice to highlight the problems.

Carers feel they should be visited every six months by someone to answer their needs, that GPs should be made more aware of mental illness, have a back-up service if a suspicion of problems arises, have more counsellors, and that there is not enough money to employ well-qualified social workers to visit everyone. A carer wishes that the churches had people who reached out of their closed communities to people in need like Jesus did outside the synagogue, and another feels she cannot ask the Church for help because she does not attend. A carer's prayer is for the strength to carry on caring for her son, and a carer, who has had many, many years of caring, feels things are much better now for carers. She acknowledges a long history of suffering for all involved, but says that they grew. A carer concludes that only those whose families or close friends have suffered and experienced firsthand the pain of mental illness show understanding and, in general, there is still, sadly, considerable stigma attached to mental health matters.

Comment

A number of conclusions can be drawn from these discussions. The first is that more literature, research, and information is needed for carers of people with mental illness. The second is that there is a need to address care in the community, especially in families where there mental ill-health and for the Church, state and voluntary bodies to work in partnership. Increased funding is needed in the state sector to provide more adequate services, especially where there is mental illness. Although there are mixed opinions as to Church funding, it would seem to need re-examining with possibly more resources for social needs, including specifically where there is mental illness. Families need more help in order to address their emotional needs and reduce tension and stress, particularly when a member has a mental illness.

Education is also a high priority for the Church and the state in order to address the problem of stigma and prejudice surrounding mental illness. Both education and training are necessary for clergy, so that these families receive pastoral care, including spiritual nourishment relevant to their needs. It is acknowledged that the needs of these families are not always recognised, or that people do not always feel able to help. Church support for carers is important and home visits where there is mental illness would seem another priority, but clergy feel over-stretched and that lay people need to be more involved. Support groups are seen as an important means of receiving mutual support, spiritual nourishment, and educational value, and need to be advertised. Equally, Church-based drop-in centres are felt to be an important resource. Good media coverage is seen as important, but needs to be positive and enlightened to help remove the stigma of mental illness.

Recommendations

- Carers and families should have their needs acknowledged and be given more support, especially where there is mental illness
- Education in both Church and the state sectors needs to be undertaken to address the issue of mental illness and help remove stigma and prejudice
- Partnerships must be built up between Church and state sectors to help address care in the community
- More positive and well-informed publicity should be carried out in respect of the role of carers, especially where there is mental illness
- Education and training for clergy regarding mental illness should be made available, so that pastoral needs of carers and families can be acknowledged and addressed, and support initiated, including, where feasible, Church-based support groups, Church-based drop-in centres and home visits. All these will need informed and trained personnel
- Resources should be re-examined and reallocated with a view to addressing these issues.

* * *

When I had finished my dissertation, it had seemed like a miracle. It had been posted without delay to my tutor who shortly afterwards wrote and congratulated me on its completion. He was delighted with it, but I would have to wait a little longer for my results to come through.

I finally received the telephone call I had been waiting for. Elizabeth had gone to the hospital and at last her baby was on the way. I had a very restless night and rang the hospital the next morning, but it would still be some time yet before the birth. Later that morning, Elizabeth telephoned me after going into the delivery room and asked would I go in. I stayed with her and Kev through the last eleven hours of a long and difficult labour and was privileged to be present at the birth of her daughter. I couldn't stop my tears as I held this tiny person, newly born, in my arms. She was beautiful. It was a wondrous occasion that words cannot quite express. I had been through so much with Elizabeth never dreaming of the day when I might hold her baby and I can't hold back my tears again as I write this.

Abbey Grace is now four months old and Elizabeth is back at work part-time as personal secretary to a divisional manager. Seven weeks after Abbey's birth, Jacqueline, too, had a baby girl, Olivia Jane, and quite a surprise for her and Dave as they were expecting a boy, but she is a joy and delight to them. We are looking forward to Christmas 1998 and Abbey's christening planned for 3rd January, 1999 at which we hope to have present all our children and our grandchildren, including the oldest two from Reading.

Susan came and listened to a talk I gave in December on carers and people with mental illness. We had a long chat afterwards. Anne makes very slow progress. I am planning a fund-raising event with the help of friends in the New Year to raise money to send Anne to Lourdes again and, hopefully, Susan with her, as they had enjoyed their first visit so much. I have also been asked to speak on the local radio station about my dissertation and while I become nervous, I always accept this sort of invitation because I feel it is an opportunity to raise awareness and educate others about these important issues.

I have learned to treasure the present and not look too far ahead, to appreciate the blessings of each day, the joy of having our daughter well after the turmoil of the past six years. We do not know whether Elizabeth's illness will return. Only God knows what the future holds.

Two weeks after Elizabeth's baby was born, I received the results of my MA degree. I had passed with distinction, but what pleased me most was receiving a distinction for my dissertation. Included in the comments was, 'this is a remarkable piece of work. The Examination Board hoped that the author would look to aspects of the work being published in some form'. This recommendation encouraged me to write my story in the hope that this book when read:

- will help in raising awareness and understanding of the trauma and stress that carers undergo when looking after a loved one with a mental illness
- will highlight carers' need for practical, emotional and spiritual support
- will give many carers hope that sometimes there can be a light at the end of the tunnel
- will help people become more aware of the depth of suffering endured by a person coping with a mental illness
- will help change attitudes towards those with mental illness, so that they might experience the love of Christ through their fellow men and women
- will help fulfill Christ's words to be spoken on the day of judgment when he will say,

'Come you whom my Father has blessed, take for your heritage the Kingdom prepared for you... for in so far as you did this to one of the least of these brothers of mine, you did it to me' (Mt.25.33:34; 40).

BIBLIOGRAPHY

Scripture and Magisterial Works

Catechism of the Catholic Church (1994) Geoffrey Chapman, London

Flannery A, ed. (1982) Vatican Council II, More Post Conciliar Documents: John Paul II (1981). *'Familiaris Consortio' The Christian Family in the Modern World*. Costello, New York.

Flannery A, ed. (1982) Vatican Council II, More Post Conciliar Documents: The Holy See (1981) *The International Year of Disabled Persons*. Costello, New York.

Flannery A, ed. (1982) Vatican Council II, More Post Conciliar Documents: Sacred Congregation for Divine Worship (1972) *'Hominum Dolores' Introduction to the Rite of Anointing and to the Pastoral Care of the Sick*. Costello, New York.

Flannery A, ed. (1987) Vatican Council II, The Conciliar and Post Conciliar Documents: Vatican II (1965). *'Apostolicam Actuositatem' Decree on the Apostolate of Lay People*. Costello, New York

Flannery A, ed. (1987) Vatican Council II, The Conciliar and Post Conciliar Documents: Vatican II (1965). *'Gaudium et Spes' Pastoral Constitution on the Church in the Modern World*. Costello, New York

Flannery A, ed. (1987) Vatican Council II, The Conciliar and Post Conciliar Documents: Vatican II (1964) *'Lumen Gentium' Dogmatic Constitution on the Church*. Costello, New York

Wansbrough, Henry (1985) *The New Jerusalem Bible*. Darton, Longman & Todd, London

Books, journals and other works

Arkless L (1995) A carer's perspective'. *Breakthrough* **1**(3): 14–15

Atkinson JM, Coia DA (1995) *Families Coping with Schizophrenia: A Practitioner's Guide to Family Groups*. John Wiley & Sons, Chichester

Bell J (1993) *Doing Your Research Project: A Guide for First-Time Researchers in Education and Social Science*, 2nd edn. Open University Press, Buckingham

Burningham S (1989) *Not on Your Own*. Penguin, London

Burton-Jones J (1992) *Caring for Carers*. Scripture Union, London

Caplin R (1993) Suicide worries. *Open Mind* **64**: 11

Card C (1995) Who cares: Walter. *Breakthrough* **1**(4): 11–12

Carson C (1992) Mental illness: support for relatives. *Nurs Stand* **6**(32): 28–31

Chiu E (1988) Caring for carers in a fragmented world. *The Way* **28**(4): 342–7

Dean M (1995) A carers perspective. *Breakthrough* **1**(3): 15–16

Edginton S (1993) Close encounters in caring. *Open Mind* **64**: 12–13

Hogman G, Pearson G (1995) *The Silent Partners: The Needs and Experiences of People who Provide Informal Care to People with a Severe Mental Illness*. National Schizophrenia Fellowship, Surrey

Hunneysett E (1994) The voice of a carer. *Priests & People* **8**(3): 11

Jee M, Reason L (1988) *Who Cares? Information and Support for the Carers of Confused People*. Health Education Authority, London

Jubilee Centre (1990) *Serving Carers: A Handbook for You and Your Church*. Jubilee Centre Publications, Cambridge

Kohner N (1992) *Caring at Home*. National Extension College, Cambridge

Kupiers L, MacCarthy B, Hurry J, Harper R (1989) Counselling the relatives of the long-term adult mentally ill: A low-cost supportive model. *Br J Psychiatry* **154**: 775–82

Ledger C (1992) *Caring for the Carers*. Kingsway Publications, Eastbourne

MacCarthy B, Kupiers L, Hurry J, Harper R, LeSage A (1989) Counselling the relatives of the long-term adult mentally ill: Evaluation of the impact on relatives and patients. *Br J Psychiatry* **154**: 768–75

McCann C (1995) *Who Cares? A Guide for All Who Care for Others*. Columba Press, Dublin

Maertens T (1964) *Bible Themes—A Source Book* II. Biblica, Bruges

Moate M, Enoch D (1990) *Schizophrenia: Voices in the Dark. Hope for Those Who Care*. Kingsway Publications, Eastbourne

Newcastle Diocesan Board for Mission and Social Responsibility (1996) *I am not an Illness*. Mental Health and Community Care, Newcastle Diocesan Board, Newcastle

Nolan P, Crawford P (1997) Towards a rhetoric of spirituality in mental health care. *J Adv Nurs* **26**: 289–94

Oglesby WB (1984) Biblical perspectives on caring for carers. *J Pastoral Care* **XXXVIII**(2): 85–90

Perrin C, Twigg J, Atkin K (1994) *Families Caring for People Diagnosed as Mentally Ill: The Literature Re-examined*. HMSO, London

Schram A (1995) Who cares. *Breakthrough* **1**(2): 13

Southwark Diocesan Board for Social Responsibility Mental Health Working Group (1994) *Travelling Together Towards Mental Health*. Southwark Diocesan Board, London

Stobbart B (1996) Carers' Needs in Middlesbrough (University of Durham: unpublished)

Swinton J, Kettles M (1997) Resurrecting the person: Redefining mental illness—a spiritual perspective. *Psychiatr Care* **4**(3): 118–21

Twigg J, Atkin K (1994) *Carers Perceived: Policy and Practice in Informal Care*. Open University Press, Buckingham

Wainright J (1997) Family Carers of Adults with Severe Mental Illness: Conceptualising Care Experience and Need (University of Durham: unpublished)

Wallace M (1996) The right to know and be heard. *Sane Talk* **Summer**: 2–5

Abbreviations

- AA Apostolicam Actuositatem
- FC Familiaris Consortio
- GS Gaudium et Spes
- HD Hominum Dolores
- LG Lumen Gentium
- CCC Catechism of the Catholic Church

Index

S

T

U

V